LOW CARB
ON THE GO

More than 80 fast, healthy

recipes – anytime, anywhere

LOW CARB ON THE GO

More than 80 fast, healthy

recipes - anytime, anywhere

Text and photography by
Sandra and Mirco Stupning

CONTENTS

CONTENTS

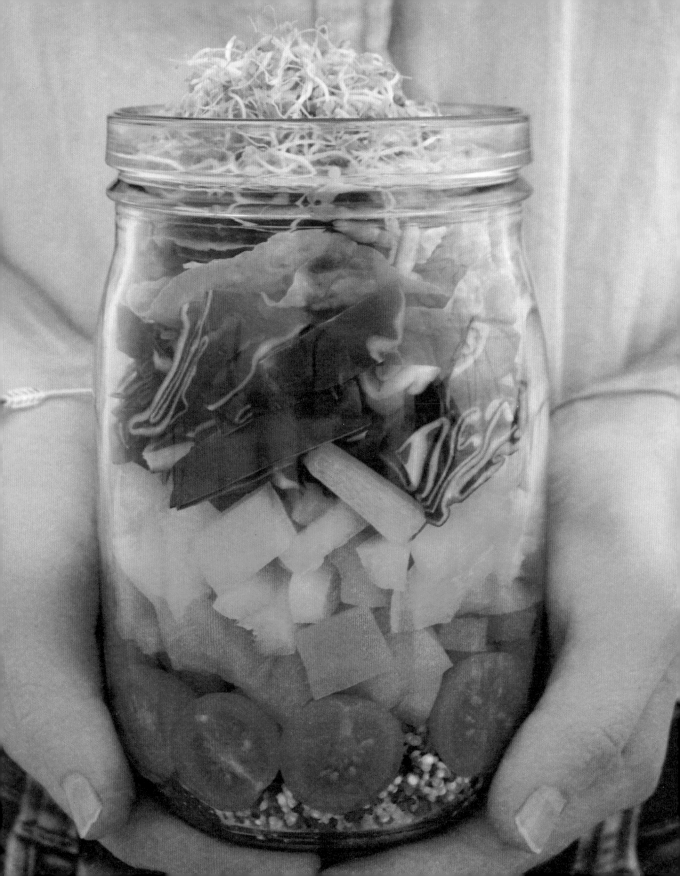

PREFACE

We are delighted that you want to prepare delicious low-carb dishes to take with you when you're out and about. We are often asked what is the easiest way to stick to a low-carb diet during lunch breaks or when you're travelling, especially since it is rare to find any low-carb takeaway options at your local sandwich bar. Our solution: prepare food at home and take it with you.

Our delicious and healthy low-carb recipes can be quickly prepared at home and the finishing touches added at work in just a few minutes. And if you have delicious ready-made food packed up for your lunch break, you won't be tempted to go and grab something else from the canteen, bakery, or supermarket. Enjoy using this book and take our healthy recipes as a source of inspiration. There is no need to follow our suggestions exactly as we have described them. Creativity and using your own favourite ingredients are invariably the best way to ensure you have fun in the kitchen and that the food you make really is to your taste.

And remember, eating together is always better than sitting alone at the table. Turn your lunch break into a communal experience. It is not just eating that is more enjoyable as a group, why not do the preparation together, too — arranging a lunch date is not unusual, but an even better idea is to meet up in the kitchen to get the food ready. It is often much easier to stick to resolutions as a group and therefore achieve pre-set goals such as eating a healthier diet. With several people to help, salads can be rustled up in no time. The food and ingredients can be agreed in advance and everyone can bring something with them, or you can take turns with your colleagues when dishes need to be prepared at home.

Our low-carb recipes will support your healthy lifestyle and boost vitality. Have lots of fun with our dishes to go.

Best wishes
SANDRA & MIRCO STUPNING

Low carb doesn't mean no carb!

The aim of a low-carb diet is to reduce, as far as possible, your consumption of poor-quality foods that are high in carbohydrates and focus instead on alternative options and healthy carbohydrates. It isn't a question of avoiding all carbohydrates; indeed, it isn't healthy for the human body to be denied carbohydrates altogether long term. If carbohydrate intake is drastically restricted, the body has to adjust to generate energy in some other way. In addition, an extreme reduction in carbohydrate consumption can have a negative impact on our health because the body is deprived of numerous important substances, particularly if this diet is followed over a longer period. This kind of radical dietary change should only be done under medical supervision. If you want to slim down healthily, you need to expend more energy than you consume, and that is best achieved through a healthy diet and exercise. The number of carbohydrates eaten should always be adjusted depending on how much physical exercise you are doing. A sensible approach is to eat fewer carbohydrates on days when you are relatively inactive than on days when you have workouts lined up. Creating a meal plan is highly recommended when losing weight.

Carbohydrates are our most important source of energy. They are needed to generate energy in the body's cells and they serve as fuel, an energy storage system, and a basic framework for our DNA and RNA, which carry our genetic information. If the body doesn't need all the energy that is provided by a meal, it converts any excess into fat stores. A diet that is low in carbohydrates, ideally combined with several exercise sessions each week, allows the body to break down any excess fat.

But the low-carb diet is not just a good choice if you wish to lose weight. Plenty of health-conscious people tend towards this lifestyle because of the focus on a varied and balanced diet and, in particular, because it avoids too many pasta products, baked goods, and highly processed or ready-made foods. Instead the emphasis is on vegetables, salads, fruits, nuts, seeds, and good-quality fats. It is not a question of banning foods, but rather placing the emphasis on choosing the right foods.

"GOOD" AND "BAD" CARBOHYDRATES

Carbohydrates vary in composition. The more complex the structure of the carbohydrate consumed, the longer the body needs to break it down and process it. The body has to break carbohydrates down into simple sugars before they can be absorbed into the bloodstream. This breakdown process, to convert molecular chains into their constituents, requires energy.

THE BUILDING BLOCKS

The basic building blocks of carbohydrates are monosaccharides (or simple sugars). In their smallest unit these consist of a single sugar molecule. Disaccharides, as the name suggests, consist of two monosaccharides joined together. Longer, partly branching sugar chains are described as oligosaccharides or polysaccharides.

Monosaccharide (simple sugars)	Disaccharide (double sugars)	Oligosaccharide (complex sugars)	Polysaccharide (complex sugars)
1 single sugar molecule	2 linked monosaccharides	3–10 linked monosaccharides	> 10 linked monosaccharides
glucose, fructose, galactose	sucrose, maltose, lactose	raffinose, stachyose, verbascose	starch, pectin, cellulose, glycogen

GOOD CARBOHYDRATES are complex carbohydrates. They consist of lots of individual sugar molecules, which are chemically bonded together in chains and are subdivided into oligosaccharides and polysaccharides. They are found, for example, in vegetables, fruits, nuts, wholegrains, and soya. The body needs longer to break down these carbohydrates, so blood sugar levels rise only slightly, the body does not produce much insulin, and the danger of storing fat in the body is low. Complex carbohydrates make you feel full for longer because the energy obtained from them remains in the body for longer. That is why eating complex carbohydrates is recommended for losing weight.

BAD CARBOHYDRATES are simple carbohydrates, which are easy to absorb. These are processed quickly by the body and enter the bloodstream swiftly. These monosaccharides and disaccharides are primarily found in processed foods containing refined sugar and white extra-fine flour. They include confectionary, pastries and pasta made from inferior quality flour, various ready meals, fast food, crisps, soft drinks, and alcoholic beverages. Simple carbohydrates are broken down swiftly by the body and don't make you feel full for long. Hunger pangs are the inevitable result.

Sugar in the blood

The most important sugar circulating in our blood is glucose – a monosaccharide. All carbohydrate compounds contained in food are broken down into individual sugar molecules by the body and can only be used once this has been done. The brain, our red blood cells, and our kidneys all rely on glucose. All other somatic cells obtain their energy primarily by metabolizing dietary fats.

The body needs more time to break down long, branching carbohydrate compounds than it does for simple compounds. This is why complex carbohydrates make us feel full for longer and allow our blood sugar levels to rise and fall gently. The reason this is important is because wild fluctuations in blood sugar levels (a blood sugar rollercoaster) cause food cravings and lapses in concentration. If blood sugar levels are constantly careering up and down, the consequence can be obesity and diabetes.

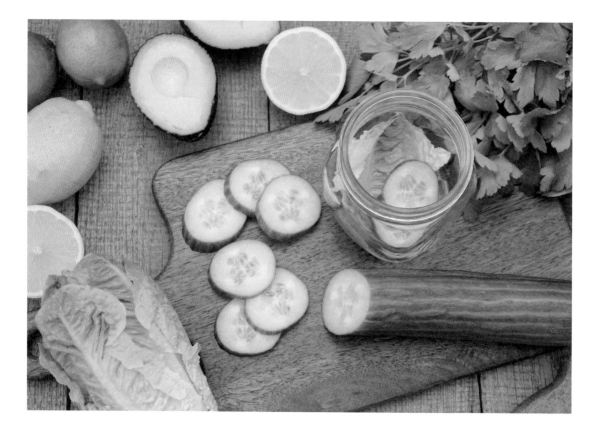

WHAT CAUSES A BLOOD SUGAR ROLLERCOASTER?

All sugar chains are broken down in the digestive organs. The resulting small sugar molecules then penetrate the cell walls and are absorbed into the blood and the blood sugar level rises. As a consequence of the rising sugar level, the brain receives a signal that the body is full and insulin is released from the pancreas. The hormone insulin allows sugar to penetrate into cells and be used as a fuel.

As soon as the sugar in our bloodstream has been absorbed by our cells, the blood sugar level falls again and the brain receives a signal that the body is hungry. At this point we often reach for something to eat again, especially sweet things (blood sugar response 1, see right). If the body is constantly exposed to this rollercoaster, this creates stress. The elevated insulin production causes a strain on the pancreas, which can result in pancreatic malfunction. In addition, the body may become resistant to insulin.

HOW CAN THIS BE AVOIDED?

It is better to eat carbohydrates that are complex in structure, with vegetables and salads top of the list. Also pulses, such as beans, lentils and peas; "activated" nuts (which have been soaked in water); wholegrains such as spelt; and pseudo grains such as buckwheat all deliver slowly digestible carbohydrates. These foods prevent blood sugar levels from rising and falling too rapidly (blood sugar response 2, see below). The dietary fibre contained in complex carbohydrates also ensures a well-regulated digestive system.

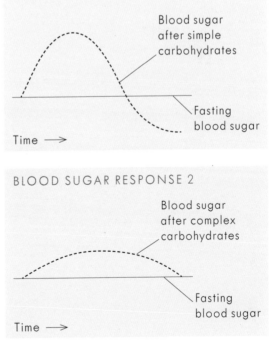

BLOOD SUGAR RESPONSE 1

Blood sugar after simple carbohydrates

Fasting blood sugar

Time ⟶

BLOOD SUGAR RESPONSE 2

Blood sugar after complex carbohydrates

Fasting blood sugar

Time ⟶

Healthy carbohydrate consumption during the day

A daily consumption of 100–150 grams of carbohydrates is ideal for the human body. The brain and nervous system require around 120 grams of carbohydrates each day; they cannot obtain energy from fats and so are dependent on glucose. If consumption is too low, the body has to take over glucose production (gluconeogenesis) itself in order to guarantee an energy supply for these organs. This isn't healthy in the long run because if you avoid carbohydrates completely, you would no longer have a balanced diet. Eating too much protein, meat, and fish is not a good foundation for a fit and healthy body. We recommend sufficient consumption of healthy carbohydrates such as vegetables and fruits, which, along with healthy carbohydrates, also contain vital nutrients and fibre.

HOW MANY MEALS SHOULD I EAT DAILY?

It is highly recommended to limit yourself to three main meals a day. This is because our digestive system functions best if we avoid constantly bombarding it with new food on top of the contents of the last meal, while this is still being processed in the digestive tract, even if this additional food is just fruit, vegetables, or a wholesome snack bar. In particular, if you are trying to lose weight, it makes sense to avoid snacks as far as possible. At first this may be really hard to stick to. Our tip: if you get peckish between meals, a glass of still water can sometimes help. Often it is not really hunger, but just thirst, food cravings, or simply habit that prompt us to start snacking.

If you really do need something to eat between meals, especially when you are initially changing over to a low-carb diet, you should stick to healthy snacks. In the morning you can chop up some fruit, or a low-carb bar is another good option. Both of these will provide energy and satisfy your cravings until the next meal, and are better than a snack containing rapidly absorbed carbohydrates such as white flour or sugar. Vegetables and nuts are suitable snacks at any time of day. Even low-carb baked goods, such as biscuits, muffins, or waffles, are great to have with you occasionally to nibble on. Other easily prepared snacks include cheese cubes, hard-boiled eggs, olives, or berries.

For each of our recipes the carbohydrate content is specified in grams. This makes it easy to plan your total carbohydrate consumption each day. The summary also specifies how many portions each recipe makes.

MORNING

Breakfast is the time when most carbohydrates should be consumed. This is because the body requires energy after its overnight rest. We recommend a portion of good carbohydrates, perhaps from a smoothie; some fromage frais or yogurt with berries; a serving of fruit, nuts, and seeds; some low-carb muesli; or low-carb bread. Since fruit is digested quickest, this should be eaten first to avoid it sitting on top of foodstuffs that take rather longer to digest. At breakfast, you should consume between 40 and 70 grams of complex carbohydrates.

MIDDAY

It is vital to make vegetables a major component of your lunchtime meal. Lots of different salads provide an ideal source of good carbohydrates. In small quantities, beans, lentils, and peas, but also quinoa and low-carb noodles can enhance the midday meal with complex carbohydrates and important nutrients. Fruit should mainly be consumed during the first half of the day and should form a smaller proportion of your intake than vegetables. For your midday meal, eat between 40 and 50 grams of carbohydrates.

EVENING

At the end of the day the body is generally winding down and it needs only a small amount of energy in the form of carbohydrates, so just a small quantity of carbohydrates should be eaten at this

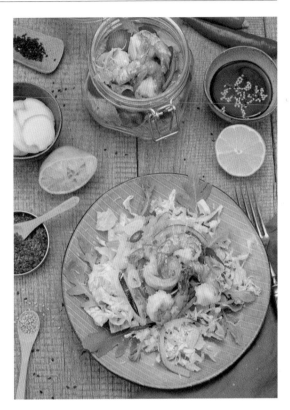

point. Salads and vegetables with a good portion of protein are ideal. Healthy sources of protein include eggs, nuts, seeds, and also mushrooms. If you opt for animal protein at supper time, you can enjoy some fish, shellfish, cheese, or meat. However, meat should not be eaten too late as the body needs several hours to digest it. Fish, on the other hand, is easier to digest and will pass through the digestive system within an hour. The recommended carbohydrate intake for the evening is no more than 30 grams.

The low carb exchange

DON'T EAT THIS	EAT THIS
pasta made from wheat or durum wheat semolina	vegetables, shirataki or low-carb noodles, wholegrain noodles in small quantities
white rice	cauliflower rice, konjac rice, wholegrain rice in small quantities
potatoes	vegetables
French fries	oven-chips made from sweet potato or courgette
bread and rolls	low-carb bread and rolls
burger buns	"oopsies" low-carb buns (see p68)
pizza	pizza with a cauliflower or low-carb flour base, low-carb pizza
white flour	flours made from nuts, linseed, coconut, hemp, chia, sesame seed or soya, wholegrains
wraps	lettuce leaves, spinach wraps, omelettes
breaded fish and meat	fish and meat without a breadcrumb coating
nuggets and other reconstituted fish and meat products	fish and meat cut as a single piece — ideally organic
ready meals, baking and sauce mixes	freshly prepared dishes
milk	plant-based "milks" such as almond, soya, oat, and coconut
ready-made muesli and breakfast cereals	home-made muesli
soft drinks	water with fresh fruits
juices	spritzers with fresh juice, tea

DON'T EAT THIS	EAT THIS
shop bought ice-cream	home-made fruit ice-cream
sweets	frozen berries and dried fruits
muesli bars	low-carb bars
cakes and biscuits	cakes and biscuits made from low-carb flours and nuts
chocolate high in sugar and with a low cocoa content	cocoa nibs, dark chocolate with a high cocoa content
chocolates and confectionery	home-made pralines from dates and nuts
latte and macchiato	coffee without milk
sugar	coconut sugar, honey, agave syrup, low-calorie sweetener such as Stevia

CHOOSE RAW NOW AND AGAIN

There are lots of benefits to eating foods raw rather than boiling, frying, or baking them. All the active ingredients are preserved and are available to our bodies in their natural form.

The most important substances in vegetables, salads, and fruit are vitamins, minerals, secondary plant substances such as glucosides, and fibre. Raw fruit and vegetables also contain enzymes. Our body requires enzymes, minerals, and vitamins for all the metabolic processes in its cells. Secondary plant substances and fibre help promote healthy digestion.

As a consequence, eating lettuce, vegetables, and fruits in their raw form is highly recommended. The greater the variety of plant-based foods consumed, the greater the range of substances obtained as a result.

Basic equipment for transporting meals

Delicious packed meals also require the right containers for transportation. Various sizes of glass jars with screwcaps (twist-off jars) or a snap-close fastening are ideal for taking meals with you. Not only are colourfully filled jars aesthetically pleasing, they are also airtight and won't leak. Glass doesn't absorb flavours and it can be filled with hot liquids without any problem. We also use circular and rectangular containers with click fasteners.

TEST FOR LEAKS

If you don't want to buy jars specially, you can use everyday food jars and containers, such as ones that once contained yogurt or jam. The most practical containers have a wide opening to make it easy to add ingredients to your meal.

Whatever kind of jar you choose, you should always test it in advance to make sure it doesn't leak. To do this, simply fill the jar with water, close it, and then stand it upside down for several minutes. Also make sure the lid doesn't open up too easily when being transported in a bag. If the glass passes the test, soak it in a tub of water for a few hours (ideally overnight) so that the label is easy to remove.

CLEAN AND SAFE

Glass jars should be sterilized before use. You can do this by washing them and putting them, without their lid, in an oven at 180°C (350°F/Gas 4) for around 10 minutes, then switch off the oven and leave the jars to cool in the closed oven. Alternatively, wash the jars and boil them for 10 minutes in a large saucepan before leaving them to cool down on a tea towel. Then the jars are ready for use. Sterilization is important for jars in which jams or spreads will be stored for long periods in the fridge. If the dish is going to be eaten promptly, it is sufficient to wash the jar before use, ideally in the dishwasher.

ALTERNATIVES TO GLASS

Unfortunately carrying glass jars is not always permitted. For example, in lots of schools and nurseries glass containers are prohibited for safety reasons. The best solution is to use a container or box made from a non-toxic material. You can also get transparent, shatterproof, odour neutral containers, which are free from harmful bisphenol A (BPA). We explicitly advise against using aluminium foil for packaging as foil can contaminate food with a worrying level of aluminium — acidic foods in particular can cause the aluminium to leach rapidly from the foil.

Icons in the book

Various icons are included on each recipe page. The icons indicate at a glance which utensils and equipment need to be taken with you for preparing the dish later at work.

	Containers: ideally glass			Hob: saucepan or frying pan
	Kettle			Cutlery: metal, wood, or even chopsticks
	Jars: large and small			Oven

WARM DISHES bring variety to your breaks. Some low-carb dishes can be eaten warm or cold as desired. We prefer to heat dishes in the oven or on the hob. Alternatively you can use a microwave oven.

THE PREPARATION TIME is subdivided into the time required at home for preparation plus baking, soaking, and so on, and the time which you will need later at work to finish preparing the dish.

NUTRITIONAL VALUES per portion are also provided in table form. The nutritional information always relates to one portion of the dish and the figures are rounded up or down to the nearest whole number.

Selecting and preparing ingredients

High-quality foods guarantee first rate enjoyment. So from the moment you go shopping you should be focused on getting top-quality, fresh produce. Our preference is to use organic ingredients.

SALAD LEAVES
should always be allowed to drain thoroughly after washing, or ideally dried using a salad spinner as this keeps the leaves fresh and crunchy for longer.

BEANS, PEAS
and other tinned foods must always be rinsed and allowed to drain thoroughly in a sieve.

EGG YOLK OR EGG WHITE
that isn't used can be kept for other dishes, such as omelettes, pancakes, or low-carb baked items.

CUCUMBER SEEDS
exude water and so are removed before taking this ingredient with you. The seeds can be used in smoothies.

HERBS
stay fresher and are more aromatic if they are chopped just before consumption.

MILK AND YOGURT
in our recipes are usually replaced by plant-based alternatives: almond, soya, or coconut milk and unsweetened natural soya yogurt.

OIL
should only be added to the dish just before eating as salad leaves in particular go mushy very quickly and won't look at all appetizing.

FROMAGE FRAIS
should not be low fat because higher-fat products have a slightly lower proportion of carbohydrates than those with a low fat content.

SALT
draws water from food and so should only be added shortly before eating. We like to use sea salt.

BEAN SPROUTS AND OTHER SHOOTS
should always be rinsed thoroughly and allowed to drain in a sieve or on some kitchen paper.

SWEETENERS
made from natural ingredients are our preferred option. These include agave syrup, coconut sugar, honey, and dates. If you would prefer to avoid carbohydrates altogether in your sugar, use a low-calorie sweetener extracted from plants such as Stevia.

LEMON AND LIME JUICE
are always freshly squeezed — we have some fruits in store at all times, ready to be squeezed.

Layering your jar

To ensure your food stays fresh and crisp until lunchtime, it is best to stick to a certain order: heavy ingredients, such as beans or cabbage, go into the jar first, which prevents lighter ingredients being crushed. Foods that exude juice, such as carrots or oranges, and ingredients that are prepared with liquid, such as quinoa, should also go into the jar first. This ensures any moisture remains at the bottom and doesn't run through all the other ingredients. Next come vegetables, then fruit, then salad. After this you can put in any meat, fish, or cheese, The uppermost layer consists of the topping, such as nuts, seeds, superfoods, or shoots, which add the finishing touch to your jar. The jar must seal tightly and be leakproof.

SEQUENCE IN THE JAR

1. Quinoa, pasta, beans
2. Vegetables
3. Fruit
4. Salad
5. Cheese, meat, fish
6. Sprouts and shoots
7. Nuts, seeds

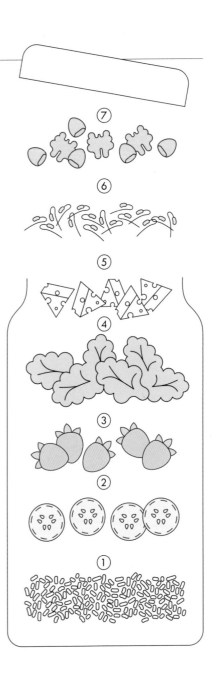

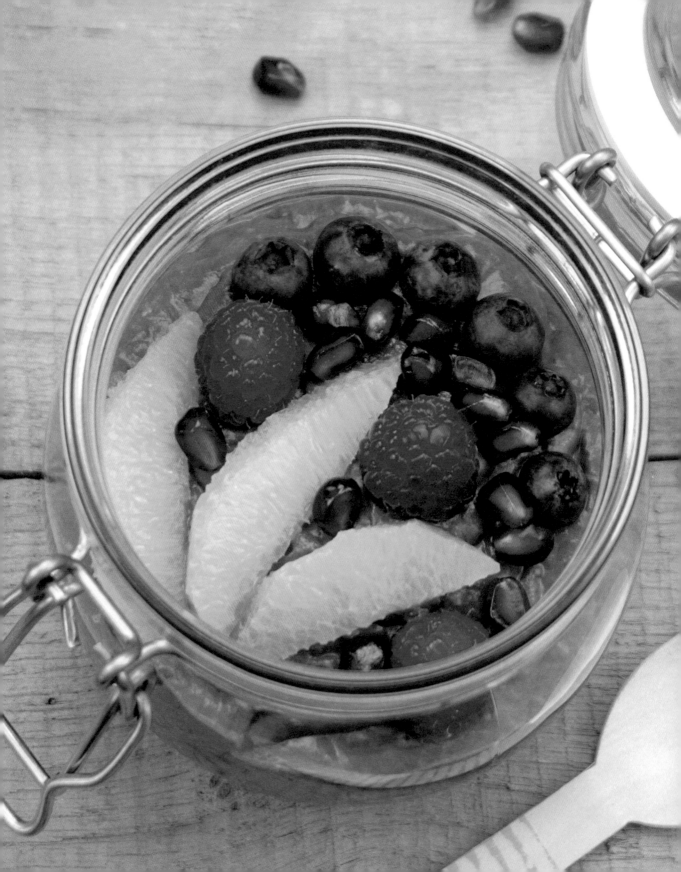

BREAKFAST

Almond milk
home-made

150g (5½oz) almonds
½ tsp lemon juice
seeds from 1 vanilla pod
pinch of salt

Wash the almonds and place them in a bowl. Cover the almonds completely with water, then add the lemon juice. Cover the bowl with cling film and leave the almonds to soak for at least 8 hours, or ideally overnight.

Drain the almonds in a sieve and rinse them again. Place the almonds, vanilla seeds, and salt in a food processor, add 400ml (14fl oz) water, and blend until the ingredients form a fine, creamy liquid. Place a large sieve over a bowl and line it with a muslin cloth. Strain the almond liquid through the cloth, doing this in several batches. If any mixture remains in the cloth, gather the corners of the cloth together above the mixture and twist firmly to squeeze the mixture out.

Pour the almond mixture into a glass bottle and seal. The almond milk can be stored in the fridge for 2–3 days. Before using, shake the bottle well to disperse the layer of fat that will have formed on the surface.

OUR TIP — You can make your own almond flour from the leftover almond purée. To do this, spread the almond mixture on a baking tray lined with baking parchment and leave to dry in a non-fan assisted oven at around 80°C (175°F/Gas low). Transfer the mixture to a food processor and blend until it is finely ground. Store the flour in the fridge.

At home	At work	Makes	Kcal	Protein	Carbs	Fat
20 min. + 8 hrs	0 mins	350ml (12fl oz)	26	1g	1g	2g

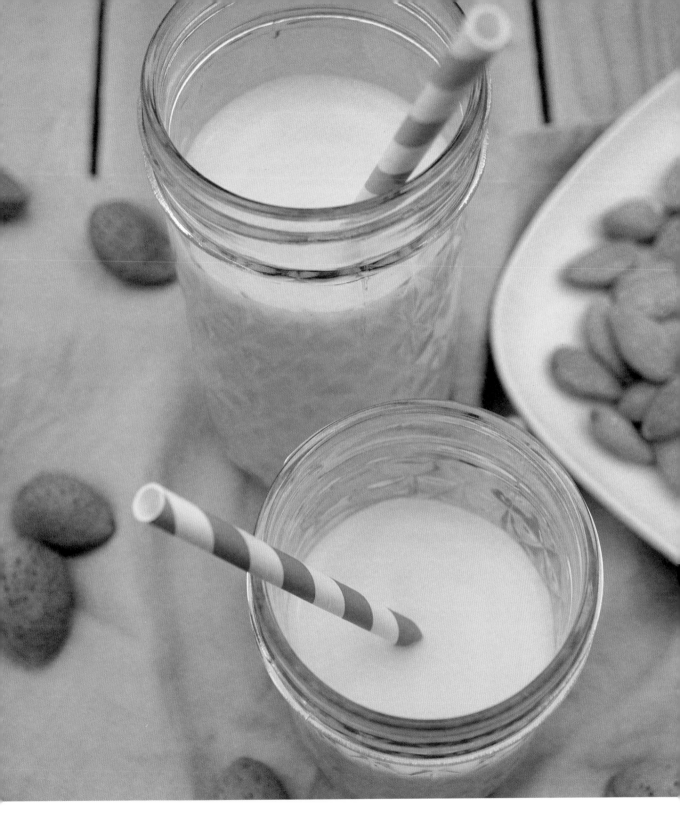

Chocolate smoothie
with avocado

½ avocado, pitted
200ml (7fl oz) almond milk
  (see p22 or shop-bought)
30g (1oz) banana, frozen
  if desired
2 tbsp raw cocoa powder
2 tsp agave syrup
cocoa nibs (optional)

Scoop out the flesh from the avocado and place in a food processor with the almond milk, banana, cocoa, and agave syrup and blend until smooth. If necessary, add a little water to obtain the desired consistency. Pour the smoothie into a jar and seal. Store in the fridge until ready to drink.

AT WORK — garnish the smoothie with cocoa nibs, if desired.

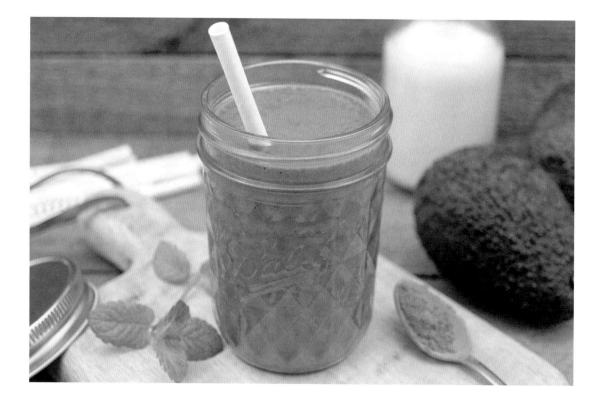

At home	At work	Serves	Kcal	Protein	Carbs	Fat
5 mins	1 min	1	317	7g	14g	20g

Strawberry chia smoothie
with almond milk

75g (2½oz) strawberries, hulled
1 tbsp yogurt
160ml (5½fl oz) almond milk
    (see p22 or shop-bought)
sliced strawberries for
    decoration (optional)
1 tbsp chia seeds

Place the strawberries, yogurt, and almond milk in a food processor and blend to a fine consistency. Decant the smoothie into a jar, adding sliced strawberries to decorate, if using. Seal the jar and store in the fridge until ready to drink. Store the chia seeds in a separate container.

AT WORK — add the chia seeds to the smoothie and shake well. Drink the smoothie straightaway as the swelling chia seeds will alter the consistency dramatically.

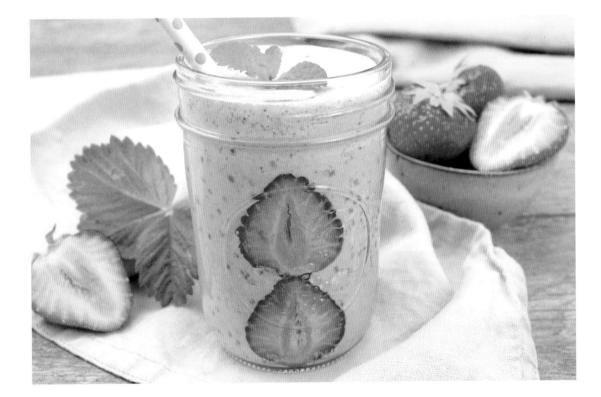

At home	At work	Serves	Kcal	Protein	Carbs	Fat
5 mins	1 min	1	107	4g	6g	6g

Cucumber shake
with dill

150g (5½oz) cucumber, chopped
4 sprigs of dill
½ small apple, cored and
    roughly chopped
100ml (3½fl oz) buttermilk
100ml (3½fl oz) soya drink
pinch of salt and freshly ground
    black pepper

Place the cucumber, dill, and apple in a food processor. Add the buttermilk, soya drink, and seasoning and blend to a fine consistency. Pour the cucumber shake into a glass bottle and seal. Store in the fridge until ready to drink.

AT WORK — decant the shake into a glass to drink.

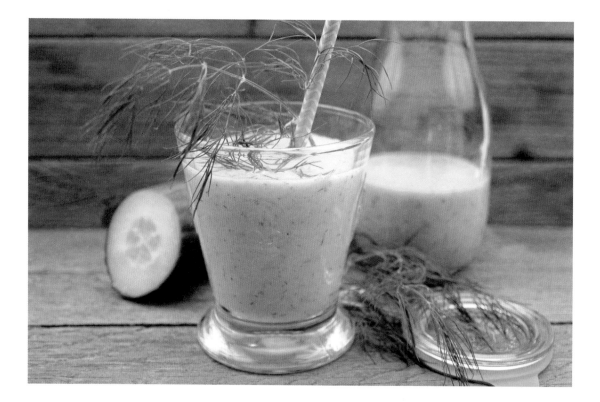

At home	At work	Serves	Kcal	Protein	Carbs	Fat
5 mins	0 min	1	135	8g	16g	4g

Orange shake
with buttermilk

130ml (4½fl oz) buttermilk
85ml (2¾fl oz) almond milk
    (see p22 or shop-bought)
1 orange, peeled and divided
    into segments
1 banana, peeled and chopped

Place the buttermilk, almond milk, orange segments, and banana pieces in a food processor and blend thoroughly. Pour the orange shake into a glass bottle and seal. Store the shake in the fridge until ready to drink.

AT WORK — decant the shake into a glass to drink.

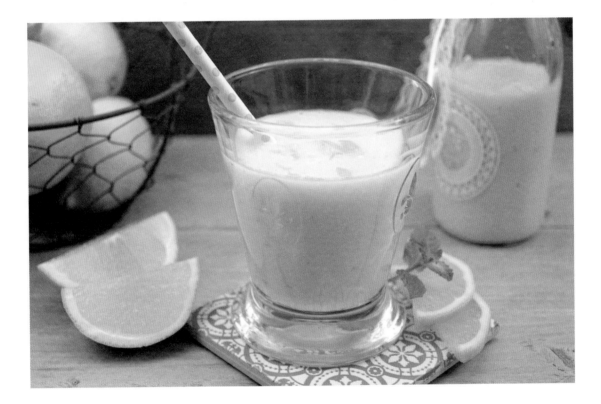

At home	At work	Serves	Kcal	Protein	Carbs	Fat
5 mins	0 min	1	173	7g	28g	3g

Mango lassi

with vanilla

½ mango, peeled, pitted, and
    cut into chunks
seeds from ½ vanilla pod
75g (2½oz) yogurt
150ml (5fl oz) almond milk
    (see p22 or shop-bought)
1 tbsp lemon juice

Place the mango in a blender beaker along with the vanilla
seeds, yogurt, almond milk, and lemon juice. Blend everything
thoroughly using a hand-held blender. Pour the mango lassi
into a glass bottle and put the lid on. Store in the fridge until
ready to drink.

AT WORK — decant the lassi into a glass to drink.

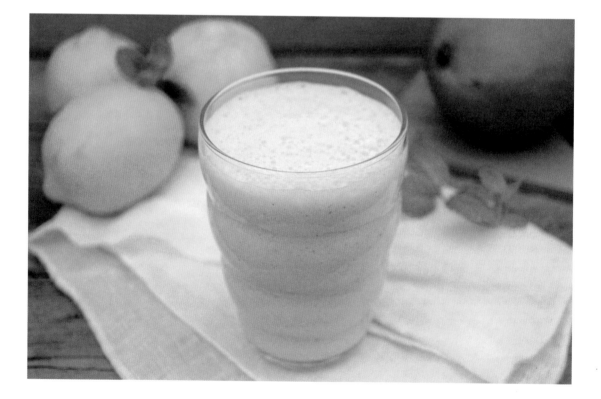

At home	At work	Serves	Kcal	Protein	Carbs	Fat
5 mins	0 min	1	136	5g	15g	4g

Mandarin citrus drink

refreshingly fruity

1 orange, divided into segments
juice of 3 mandarins
1 tbsp lemon juice

Place the orange segments in a blender beaker along with the mandarin and lemon juice. Add 200ml (7fl oz) water and blend until smooth. Pour into a jar and seal with the lid.

OUR TIP — depending on the time of year, this can be enjoyed either as a cold refreshment or heated for a warming drink.

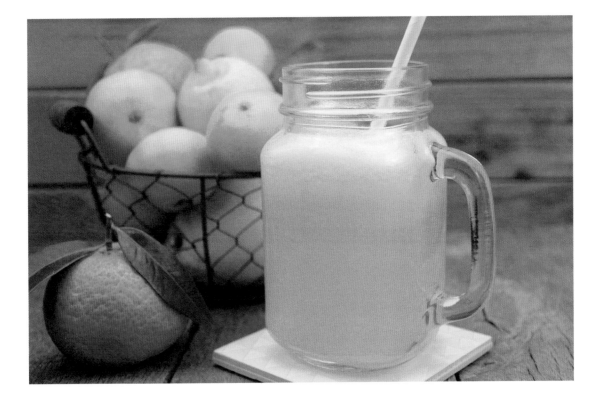

At home	At work	Serves	Kcal	Protein	Carbs	Fat
5 mins	0 min	1	80	1g	16g	0g

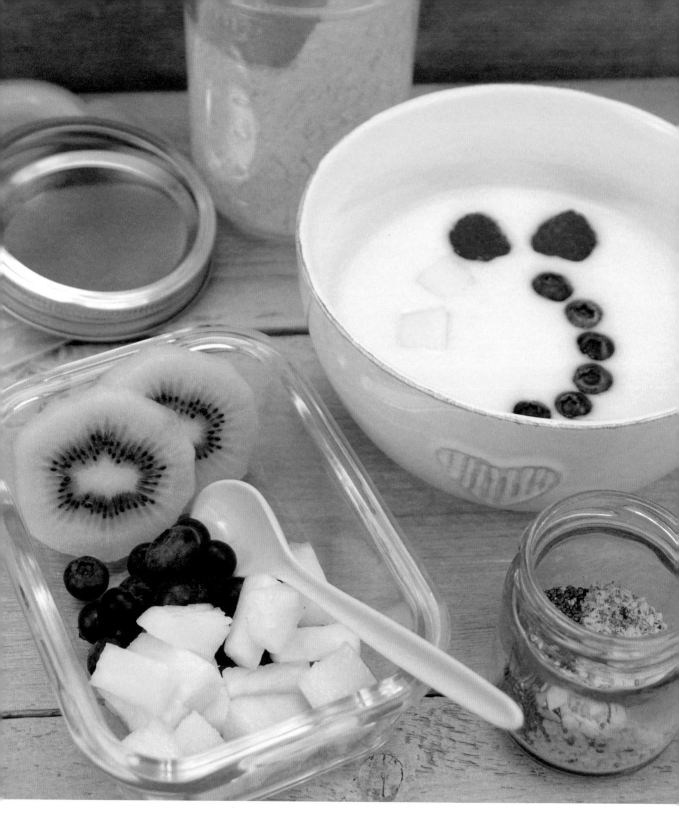

Coconut bowl
piña colada style

FOR THE SMOOTHIE

100g (3½oz) pineapple, peeled,
   cored, and chopped
3½ tbsp coconut milk
4 tbsp yogurt
agave syrup (optional)

FOR THE TOPPING

2 raspberries
1 tbsp blueberries
1 tbsp pineapple pieces
2 slices of kiwi
2 small pieces of mango
1 tsp chia seeds
1 tsp coconut flakes
2 tbsp ground almonds
edible flowers, for example,
   violas (optional)

To make the smoothie, place the pineapple pieces in a food processor with the coconut milk and yogurt and blend until smooth. If desired, sweeten the smoothie with agave syrup then quickly blend everything together again.

To remove the pineapple fibres, strain the smoothie through a sieve into an airtight jar and seal. Store the smoothie in the fridge until ready to drink.

Put all the fruit for the topping into a container, then put the chia seeds, coconut flakes, ground almonds, and edible flowers, if using, in a separate container.

AT WORK — pour the smoothie into a bowl and decorate with the topping ingredients.

At home	At work	Serves	Kcal	Protein	Carbs	Fat
10 mins	5 min	1	415	12g	25g	27g

Green smoothie bowl
with goji berries

FOR THE SMOOTHIE
½ avocado, pitted
50g (1¾oz) spinach leaves,
    coarse stems removed
30g (1oz) banana, frozen

FOR THE TOPPING
1 tsp goji berries, chopped
1 tsp blueberries
1 small piece of avocado
1 small piece of banana
2 spinach leaves (optional)
½ tsp white sesame seeds

For the smoothie, scrape the flesh from the avocado skin using a spoon. Place the spinach, avocado, banana, and 100ml (3½fl oz) water in a food processor and blend until smooth. Pour the smoothie into an airtight container and seal. Store in the fridge until ready to serve.

Put all the ingredients for the topping into a separate container.

AT WORK — pour the smoothie into a bowl and scatter over the ingredients for the topping.

OUR TIP — this looks particularly decorative if you cut stars or other shapes out of the avocado and banana, or even from the spinach leaves if you prefer.

At home	At work	Serves	Kcal	Protein	Carbs	Fat
10 mins	2 min	1	175	3 g	13 g	11 g

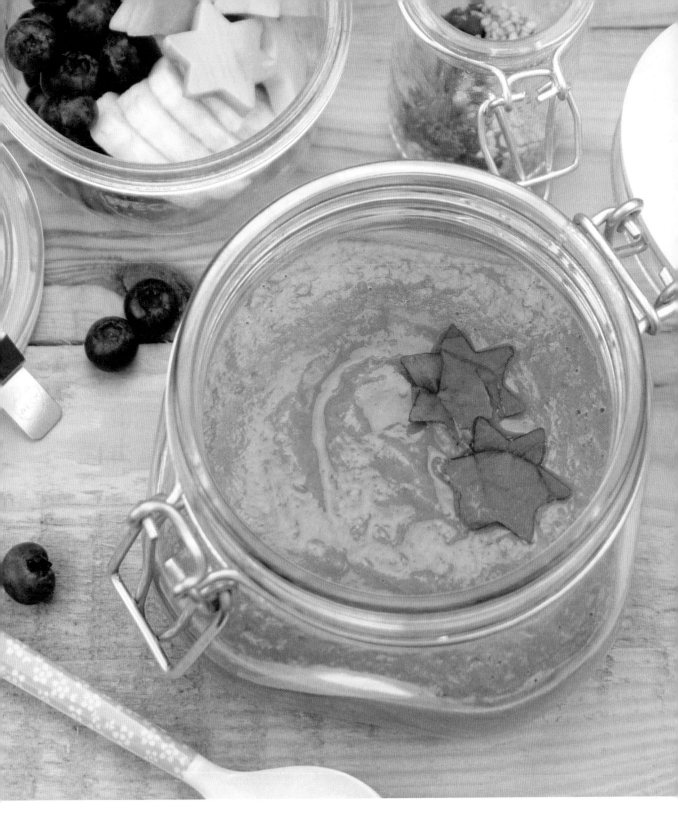

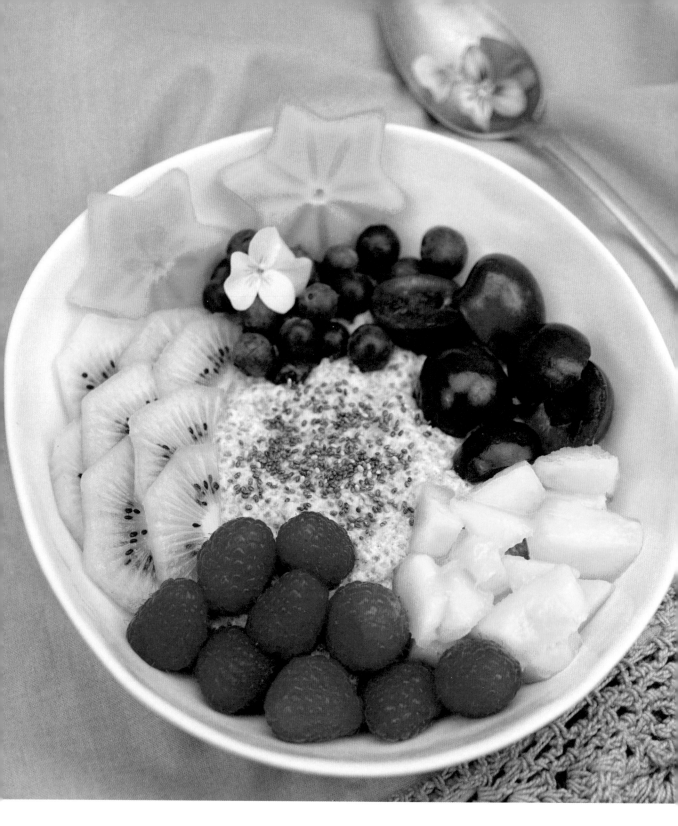

BREAKFAST

Chia breakfast bowl

with fruit

FOR THE BREAKFAST BOWL
20g (¾oz) chia seeds
100ml (3½fl oz) coconut milk

FOR THE TOPPING
2 tbsp raspberries
2 tbsp blueberries
1 kiwi, peeled and sliced
3 sweet cherries, pitted
    and halved
¼ persimmon, peeled and
    sliced, or cut into star shapes
1 tbsp mango pieces
edible flowers, for example,
    violas (optional)

To make the breakfast bowl, combine the chia seeds with the coconut milk in a bowl and leave to swell.

Transfer the chia mixture into an airtight container and seal. Put the fruits for the topping into a separate container. Store the chia mixture, fruits, and edible flowers (if using) in the fridge until ready to serve.

AT WORK — pour the chia mixture into a bowl and decorate with the fruit topping and edible flowers, if desired.

At home	At work	Serves	Kcal	Protein	Carbs	Fat
15 mins	1 min	1	385	7g	22g	26g

Choco chia bowl
with fruit

FOR THE SMOOTHIE
½ avocado, pitted
20g (¾oz) banana, frozen
2 tbsp raw cocoa powder
1 tbsp chia seeds
1–2 tsp agave syrup
100ml (3½fl oz) almond milk
   (see p22 or shop-bought)

FOR THE TOPPING
¼ orange, peeled, and
   divided into segments
1 tbsp blueberries
1 tbsp raspberries
1 tbsp pomegranate seeds
mint or lemon balm leaves
   (optional)

Scrape out the flesh from the avocado skin using a spoon.

Place the avocado flesh in a food processor along with the banana, cocoa powder, chia seeds, agave syrup, and almond milk and blend everything until smooth. If required, add a little water to obtain the desired consistency. Transfer the smoothie to an airtight container and seal. Store in the fridge until ready to serve.

For the topping, put the orange segments, blueberries, raspberries, and pomegranate seeds in a container and, if using, put the mint or lemon balm leaves into a separate container.

AT WORK — transfer the choco chia smoothie into a bowl and decorate with the topping. Garnish with mint or lemon balm leaves, if desired.

At home	At work	Serves	Kcal	Protein	Carbs	Fat
5 mins	2 min	1	445	12g	19g	34g

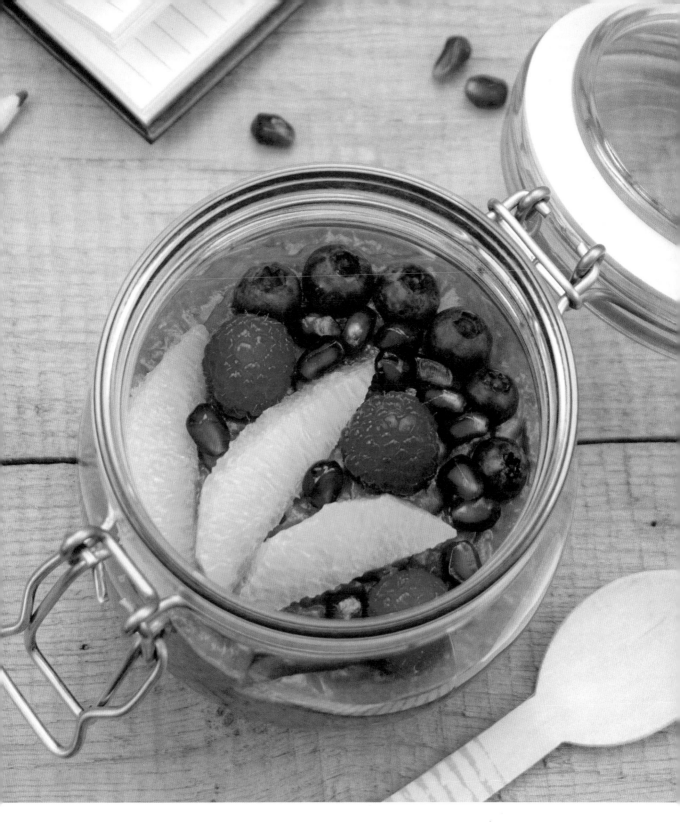

BREAKFAST

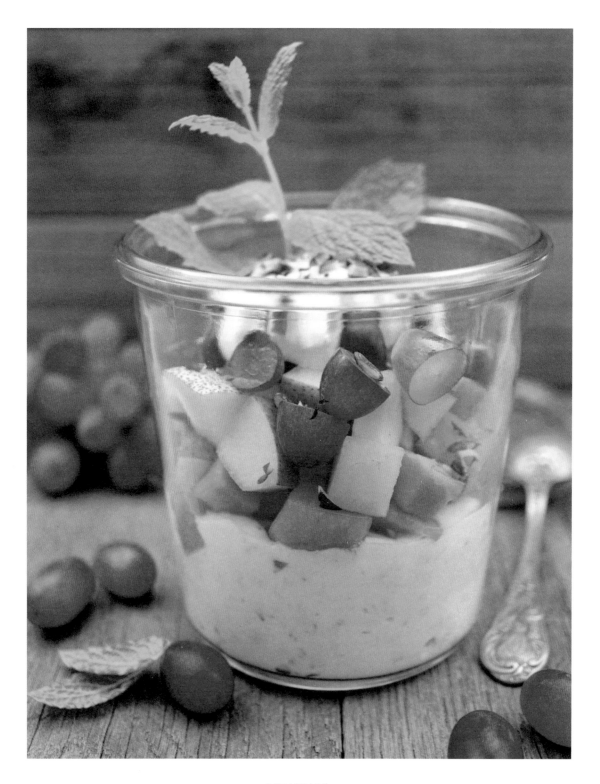

BREAKFAST

Papaya pear fromage frais

with pumpkin seeds

150g (5½oz) full-fat fromage frais
1 tbsp spelt flakes
1 tbsp mint, chopped
75g (2½oz) papaya, cored and
    chopped into bite-size pieces
¼ pear, cored and cut into cubes
handful of grapes (red or white,
    as preferred), halved
1 tbsp pumpkin seeds, coarsely
    chopped
sprig of mint, to garnish (optional)

Place the fromage frais, spelt flakes, and mint together in a bowl and stir until combined.

Put the mixture into a jar, setting aside 1 tablespoon for decoration. Layer the papaya, pear, and grapes on top. Add a blob of the remaining fromage frais mixture and scatter with the pumpkin seeds. Garnish with the sprig of mint, if desired. Place the lid on the jar and store the papaya and pear fromage frais in the fridge until ready to serve.

At home	At work	Serves	Kcal	Protein	Carbs	Fat
5 mins	0 min	1	358	18g	31g	18g

Lime mandarin fromage frais

with superfoods

FOR THE CHIA GEL
1 tsp ground dried dandelion
   leaves (available from
   health-food stores)
1 tbsp chia seeds
1 tsp mint, chopped
1–2 tsp agave syrup

FOR THE FROMAGE FRAIS
juice and zest of 1 organic lime,
   plus slice of lime, to garnish
   (optional)
250g (9oz) full-fat fromage frais
juice of 1 mandarin
dash of agave syrup

FOR THE SUPERFOOD
TOPPING
½ tsp sunflower seeds
½ tsp goji berries
½ tsp pumpkin seeds
½ tsp cocoa nibs
½ tsp hemp seeds
½ tsp pistachio kernels

To make the chia gel, place 100ml (3½fl oz) water, 2 tbsp of lime juice from the fromage frais mixture, and the dandelion leaves in a bowl and stir to combine. Mix in the chia seeds and leave to swell for at least 10 minutes. Stir in the mint and agave syrup.

In a separate bowl, stir together the fromage frais, the remaining lime juice, and the mandarin juice. Mix in the grated lime zest and agave syrup.

To make the superfood topping, roughly chop all the ingredients then mix them together in a bowl. Transfer the chia gel to a jar, add the fromage frais mixture and, if desired, garnish with a slice of lime. Finally, top with the chopped superfoods. Place the lid on the jar and store in the fridge until ready to serve.

At home	At work	Serves	Kcal	Protein	Carbs	Fat
20 mins	0 min	1	504	26g	32g	30g

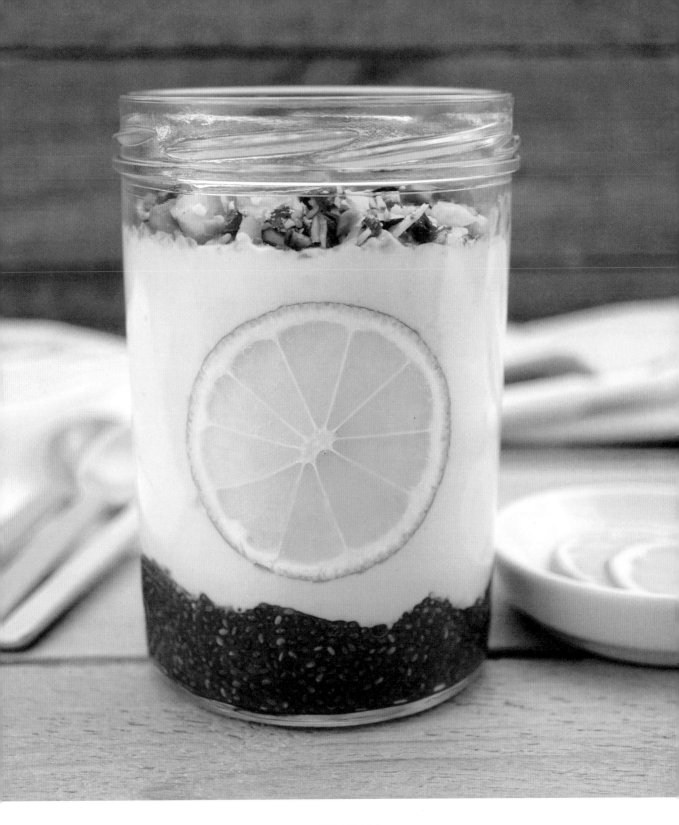

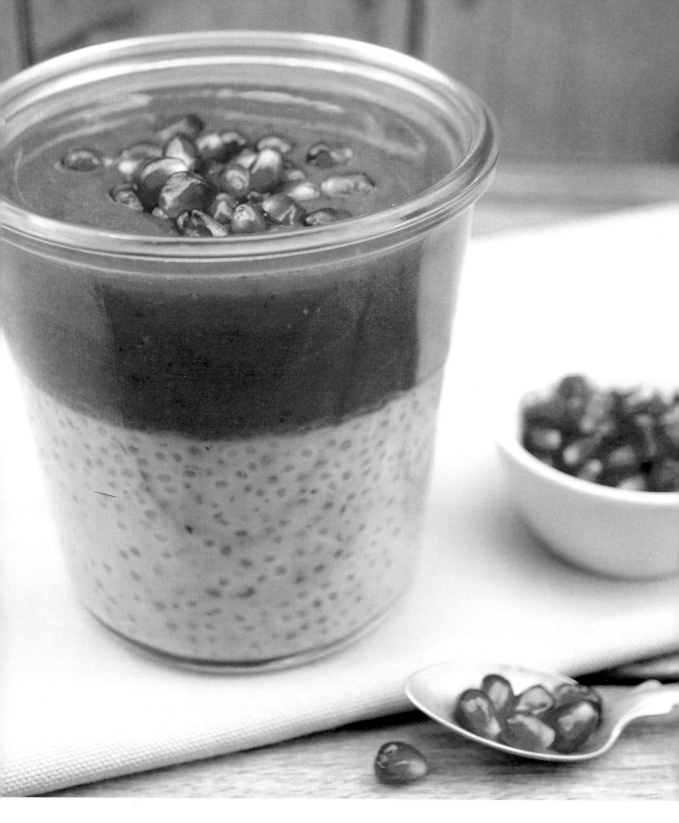

Chia pudding with berry purée
and pomegranate seeds

1 tbsp chia seeds
150g (5½oz) mixed berries
    (fresh or frozen)
1 tbsp low-calorie sweetener,
    such as Stevia
200g (7oz) yogurt
1 tbsp pomegranate seeds

Mix the chia seeds with 130ml (4½fl oz) water in a bowl and leave to swell for at least 10 minutes. Purée the berries in a high-sided container using a hand-held blender (there is no need to defrost frozen berries).

Stir the sweetener into the yogurt. Combine the yogurt mixture with the chia gel, stirring well.

Transfer the chia pudding to a jar. Top with the berry purée and scatter with pomegranate seeds. Place the lid on the jar and store the chia dessert in the fridge until ready to serve.

At home	At work	Serves	Kcal	Protein	Carbs	Fat
15 mins	0 min	1	260	12g	18g	9g

Fromage frais muesli
with melon

1 tbsp oats
100g (3½oz) yogurt
100g (3½oz) full-fat fromage frais
½ small apple, cored and
   chopped into bite-size chunks
1 orange, peeled, divided into
   segments, then chopped into
   small pieces
60g (2oz) Galia melon, flesh
   removed and chopped into
   bite-size chunks
1 tbsp linseed
1 tsp cashews, roughly chopped

Place the oats in a bowl with 2 tbsp water, stir, and leave to soak for 5–10 minutes then pour away any excess water. Stir the yogurt and fromage frais into the oats.

Combine all the fruit pieces in a bowl with the linseed and cashew nuts.

Transfer the yogurt and fromage frais mixture into an airtight jar and arrange the fruit on top. Place the lid on the jar and store the muesli in the fridge until ready to serve.

At home	At work	Serves	Kcal	Protein	Carbs	Fat
10 mins	0 min	1	327	17g	25g	16g

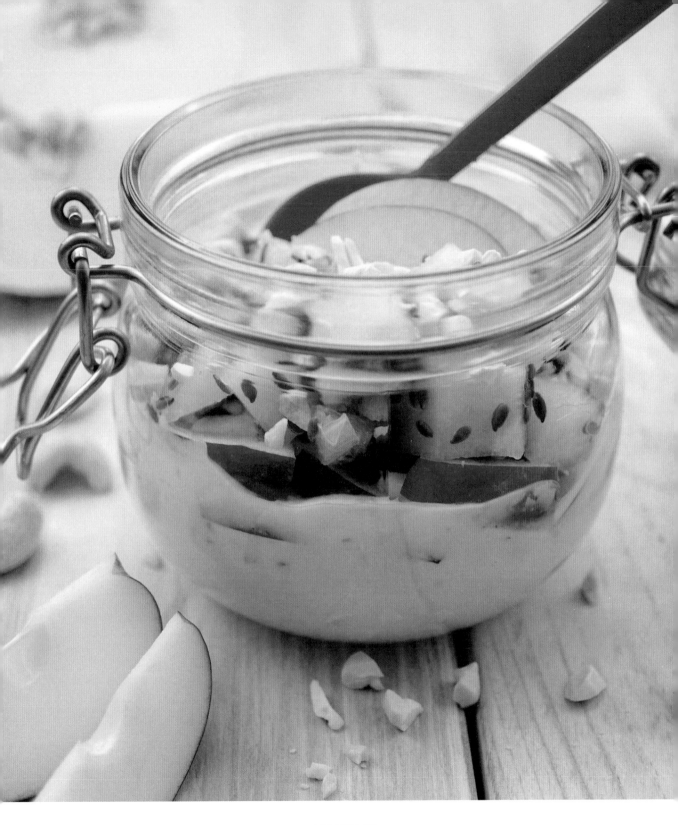

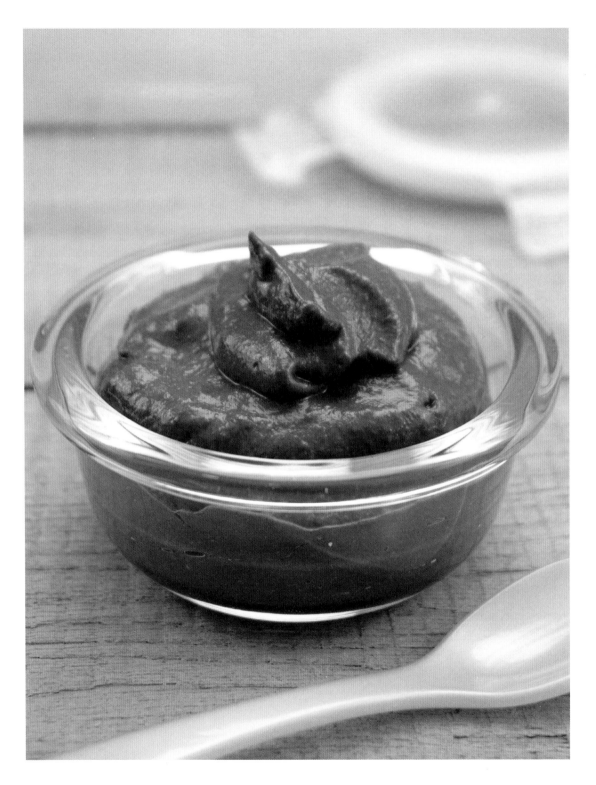

BREAKFAST

Chocolate pudding
extra creamy

1 avocado, halved and pitted
15g (½oz) raw cocoa powder
2 dates, pitted
80ml (2½fl oz) almond milk
   (see p22 or shop-bought)

Use a spoon to scoop the flesh from the avocado skin, then add to a high-sided blender beaker along with the cocoa powder, dates, and almond milk.

Use a hand-held blender to purée the pudding ingredients to a fine and creamy consistency. Transfer to a lidded jar. Store the pudding in the fridge until ready to serve.

At home	At work	Serves	Kcal	Protein	Carbs	Fat
5 mins	0 min	1	314	6g	9g	28g

Strawberry bowl
with avocado

1 avocado, halved and pitted
1 tsp lime juice
2 tsp chia seeds
60g (2oz) strawberries, hulled
85g (3oz) yogurt
30g (1oz) mango

Peel one half of the avocado and slice into strips, then drizzle with the lime juice. Put the avocado slices, chia seeds, and 1 strawberry into separate containers. Scrape the remaining avocado flesh from the skin and blend in a food processor with the remaining strawberries, the yogurt, and the mango until the mixture is a fine consistency. Store in a container in the fridge.

AT WORK — transfer the mixture into a bowl and garnish with the avocado slices, strawberries, and chia seeds.

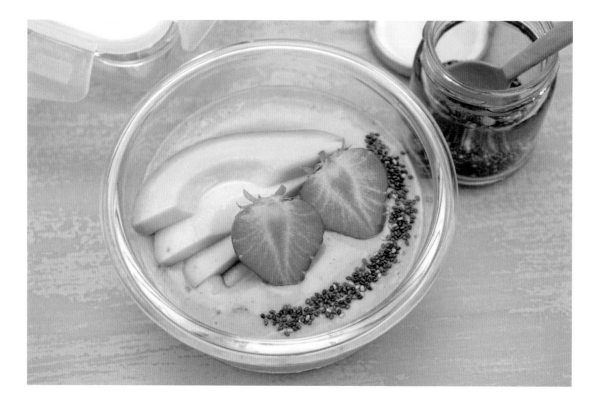

At home	At work	Serves	Kcal	Protein	Carbs	Fat
5 mins	1 min	1	405	8g	10g	35g

Chia pick-me-up
with turmeric

2 tbsp chia seeds, plus a few
  more, to garnish
100ml (3½fl oz) soya drink
50g (1¾oz) full-fat fromage
  frais, plus 1 tbsp, to garnish
1 tsp ground turmeric
1 tbsp lemon juice
dash of agave syrup
½ kiwi, peeled and sliced

Place the chia seeds and soya drink in a bowl, stir, and leave
the seeds to swell for at least 10 minutes. Stir in the fromage
frais, turmeric, lemon juice, and agave syrup. Transfer the chia
dessert to a jar, adding some whole kiwi slices as desired and
setting aside the remaining slices. Garnish with 1 tbsp fromage
frais and a few chia seeds. Halve the remaining kiwi slices and
stick them into the top. Seal the jar and store your pick-me-up
in the fridge until required.

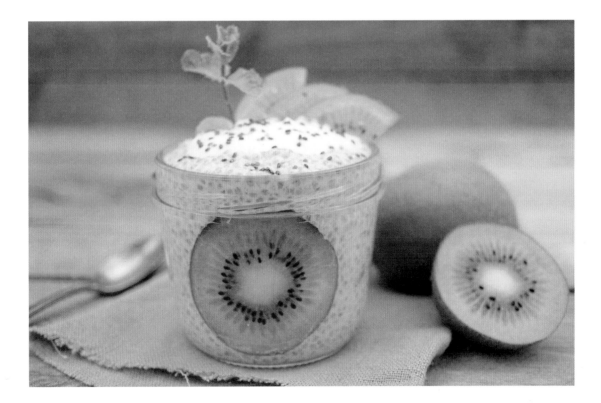

At home	At work	Serves	Kcal	Protein	Carbs	Fat
15 mins	0 min	1	409	14g	14g	26g

Coconut muesli

with a crunch

100g (3½oz) coconut flakes
30g (1oz) sunflower seeds
50g (1¾oz) chopped almonds
25g (scant 1 oz) walnuts, chopped
25g (scant 1 oz) coconut flour
2 egg whites
1 tbsp protein powder (coconut)
1 tsp low-calorie sweetener,
    such as Stevia

Preheat the oven to 130°C (250°F/Gas ½). Line a baking tray with baking parchment. Mix all the ingredients with 4 tsp water. Spread the mixture over the baking parchment and bake in the centre of the oven for 20–30 minutes, until pale gold in colour, stirring the mixture two or three times during this period. Remove from the oven, leave to cool, and store in an airtight jar.

OUR TIP — this coconut muesli tastes fantastic with almond milk (see p22).

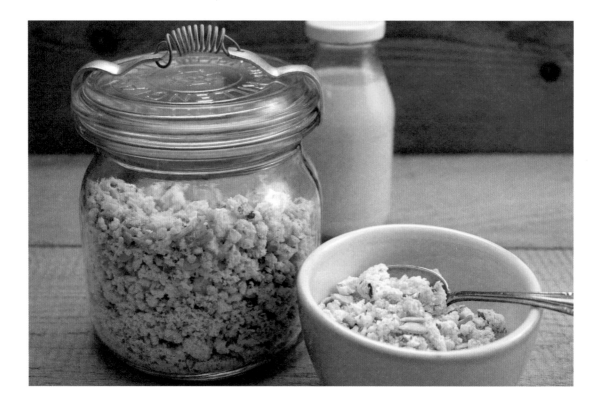

At home	At work	Serves	Kcal	Protein	Carbs	Fat
40 mins	0 min	6	240	8g	5g	20g

Revitalizing muesli

nutty and wholesome

1 tbsp coconut oil
1½ tbsp honey
20g (¾oz) flaked almonds
25g (scant 1 oz) oats
10g (¼oz) coconut flour
10g (¼oz) ground almonds
½ tsp vanilla powder (or seeds
   from ½ vanilla pod)
pinch of salt

Preheat the oven to 140°C (275°F/Gas 1). Line a baking tray with baking parchment. Melt the oil with the honey in a pan over a low heat. Crumble the flaked almonds and combine with the oats, coconut flour, ground almonds, vanilla, salt, and the oil mixture. Bake the muesli on the tray in the centre of the oven for 10 minutes. Reduce the temperature to 100°C (212°F), stir the muesli, and bake for a further 5–10 minutes, until golden brown. Leave to cool and store in an airtight jar.

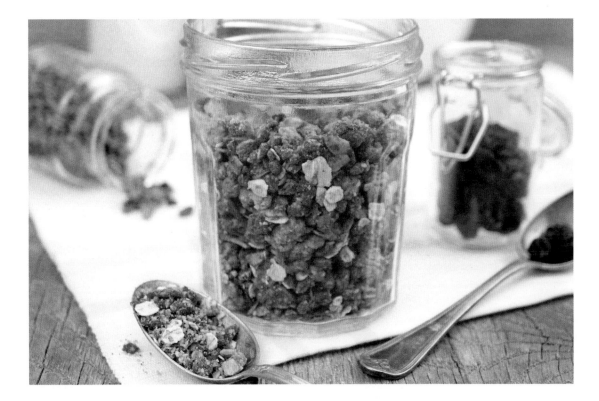

At home	At work	Serves	Kcal	Protein	Carbs	Fat
20 mins	0 min	3	170	4g	11g	12g

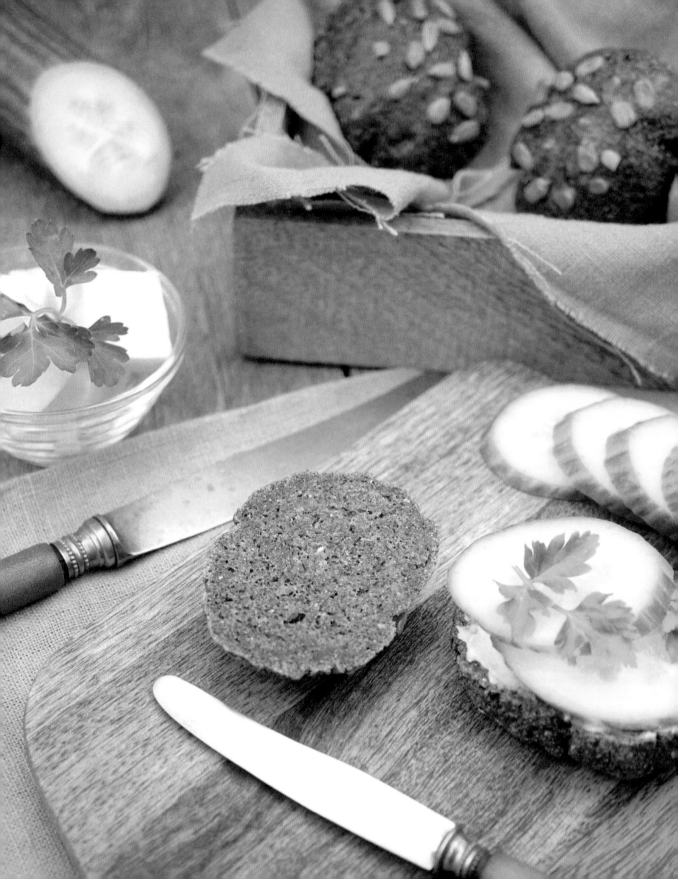

BREADS AND

SPREADS

Blueberry vanilla spread

fruity and delicious

75g (2½oz) blueberries
   (fresh or frozen)
2 tbsp chia seeds
1 tsp vanilla powder
2 tbsp agave syrup

Place the blueberries in a high-sided container and use a hand-held blender to purée them thoroughly (frozen berries can be blended without defrosting). Stir in the chia seeds, vanilla powder, and agave syrup with a spoon. Leave the spread to stand for at least 30 minutes. Transfer to a lidded jar. Store in the fridge for up to 1 week.

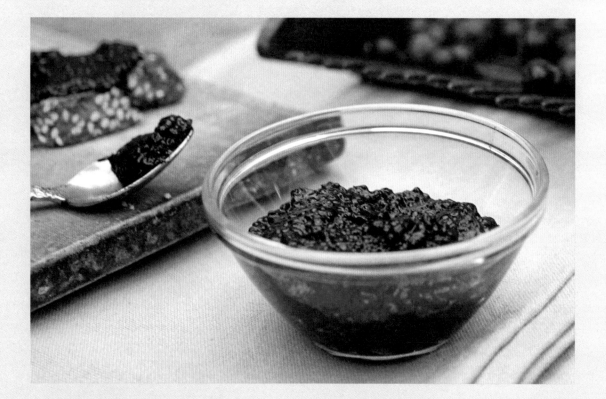

At home	At work	Serves	Kcal	Protein	Carbs	Fat
5 + 30 mins	0 min	5	40	1g	5g	1g

Raspberry chia spread

a taste of summer

75g (2½oz) raspberries
   (fresh or frozen)
2 tbsp chia seeds
1 tbsp agave syrup

Place the raspberries in a high-sided container and use a hand-held blender to purée them thoroughly (frozen berries can be blended without defrosting). Stir in the chia seeds and syrup with a spoon. Leave the spread to stand for at least 30 minutes. Transfer to a lidded jar. Store in the fridge for up to 1 week.

OUR TIP — leave the spread to stand overnight before using.

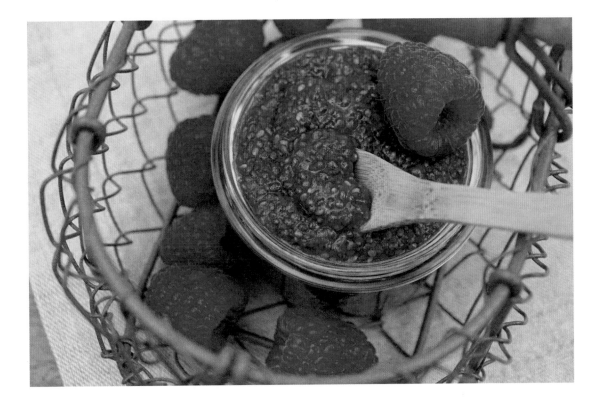

At home	At work	Serves	Kcal	Protein	Carbs	Fat
5 + 30 mins	0 min	5	30	1g	3g	1g

Cashew butter

alternative to butter

100g (3½oz) cashews
1 tbsp sunflower oil

Lightly toast the cashew nuts in a pan without any oil, turning them regularly.

Place the toasted cashews in a high-sided container together with the sunflower oil and use a hand-held blender to purée them as finely as possible.

Transfer the cashew butter to a lidded jar. Store in the fridge for up to 4 weeks.

At home	At work	Serves	Kcal	Protein	Carbs	Fat
5 mins	0 min	5	135	3g	6g	10g

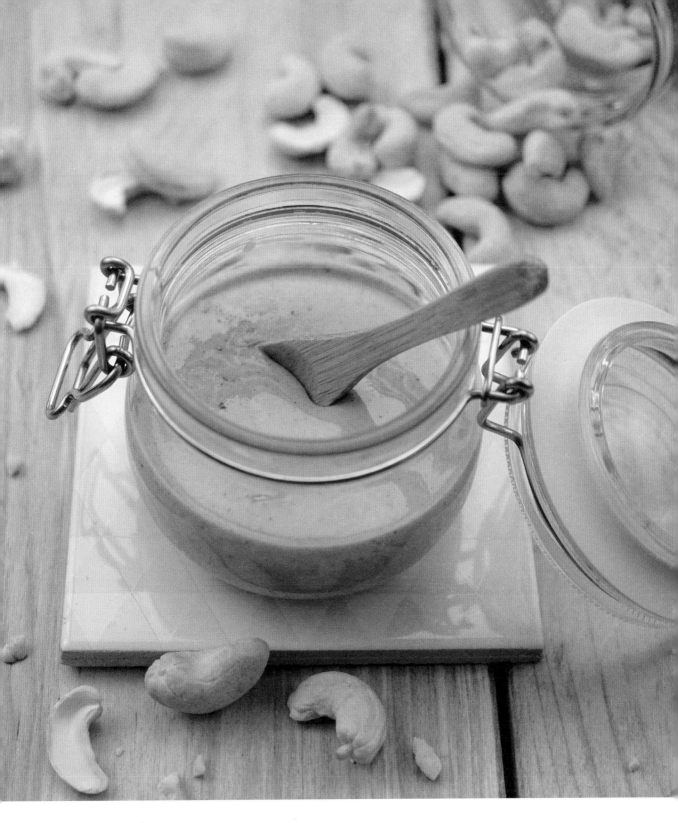

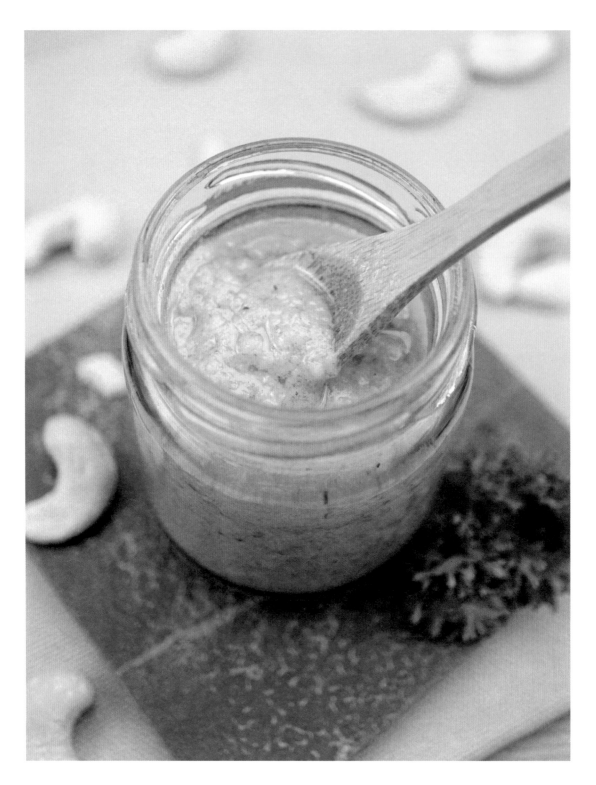

Cashew citrus cream

zesty and aromatic

40g (1¼oz) cashews
salt and freshly ground
    black pepper
1–2 sprigs parsley (curly
    or flat leaf, as desired)
3 mint leaves
2 tbsp olive oil
1 tbsp orange juice
1 tsp lemon juice
1 tsp agave syrup
1 tsp organic lemon zest

Place the cashews in a bowl with 90ml (3fl oz) water and a pinch of salt and leave to soak for at least 1 hour. Then strain off the water in a sieve, rinse the cashews, and leave to drain.

Transfer the cashews to a high-sided container and add the herbs, followed by the olive oil, orange juice, lemon juice, agave syrup, lemon zest, and a pinch of salt and pepper. Using a hand-held blender, purée the ingredients thoroughly.

Decant the cashew citrus cream into a lidded jar. Store in the fridge for several days.

At home	At work	Serves	Kcal	Protein	Carbs	Fat
5 + 60 mins	0 min	5	100	1g	3g	9g

Cucumber radish fromage frais
with beetroot shoots

100g (3½oz) full-fat fromage frais
85g (3oz) cucumber, peeled and
    cut into cubes
4 radishes, finely chopped
2 sprigs of flat leaf parsley,
    leaves removed and finely
    chopped
1 tbsp beetroot shoots
salt and freshly ground
    black pepper

Place the fromage frais, cucumber, radish, and parsley in a bowl, combine, and season with salt and pepper. Transfer the fromage frais mixture to a jar. Either add the shoots directly on top or pack them separately. Put the lid on the jar and store the spread in the fridge until ready to serve.

AT WORK — stir the fromage frais thoroughly then spread it on some low-carb rolls (recipe see p77), or similar. If you packed the shoots separately, scatter these over the fromage frais.

At home	At work	Serves	Kcal	Protein	Carbs	Fat
5 mins	1 min	1	151	9g	8g	9g

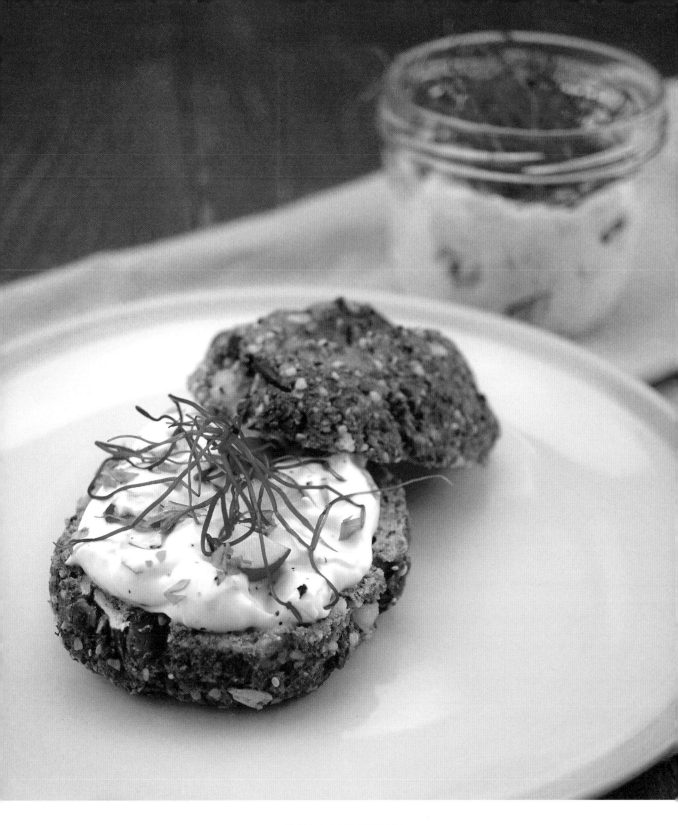

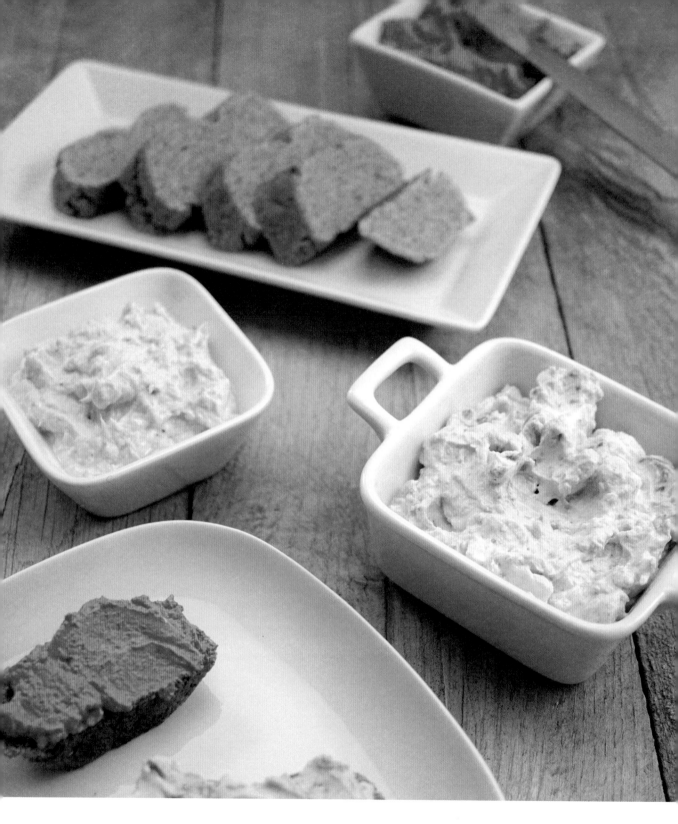

Three kinds of dips

for all your sandwich breaks

BEETROOT DIP

30g (1oz) cooked beetroots
85g (3oz) full-fat cream cheese
1 splash lemon juice
pinch of low-calorie sweetener,
   such as Stevia
salt and freshly ground
   black pepper

Peel and chop the beetroots, then purée using a hand-held blender. Stir in the cream cheese, lemon juice, and the sweetener. Season the dip to taste.

At home	At work	Serves	Kcal	Protein	Carbs	Fat
5 mins	0 min	4	235	6g	15g	20g

TUNA FISH DIP

25g (scant 1 oz) tinned tuna
½ shallot, finely chopped
1 tsp capers, chopped
60g (2oz) full-fat cream cheese
1 tsp lemon juice
salt and freshly ground
   black pepper

Drain the tuna and squeeze it out using kitchen paper. Place the tuna fish and shallots in a high-sided container and use a hand-held blender to process them to a lumpy consistency. Add the cream cheese, capers, and lemon juice to the tuna purée, and stir until well combined. Season the dip to taste.

At home	At work	Serves	Kcal	Protein	Carbs	Fat
5 mins	0 min	4	200	11g	2g	16g

TOMATO DIP

30g (1oz) sundried tomatoes in oil
60g (2oz) full-fat cream cheese
splash of lime juice
salt and freshly ground
   black pepper

Drain and chop the tomatoes, then place them in a high-sided container and use a hand-held blender to process them to a lumpy consistency. Stir in the cream cheese and lime juice. Season the dip to taste.

At home	At work	Serves	Kcal	Protein	Carbs	Fat
5 mins	0 min	4	220	6g	7g	18g

Goat's cheese spread

Mediterranean style

2 sprigs of rosemary, leaves
    picked and roughly chopped
sprig of thyme, leaves picked
    and roughly chopped
5 sundried tomatoes in oil,
    finely chopped
100ml (3½fl oz) olive oil
1 tsp dried basil
40g (1¼oz) goat's cheese,
    sliced into two discs

Put the olive oil into a jar with the rosemary, thyme, basil, and tomatoes, then add the goat's cheese discs.

Place the lid on the jar and store in the fridge until ready to serve. The cheeses will keep for up to approximately 4 weeks in the fridge, provided they are always well covered in oil.

OUR TIP — ideally leave the goat's cheese to infuse overnight.

At home	At work	Serves	Kcal	Protein	Carbs	Fat
5 mins	0 min	2	140	5g	4g	11g

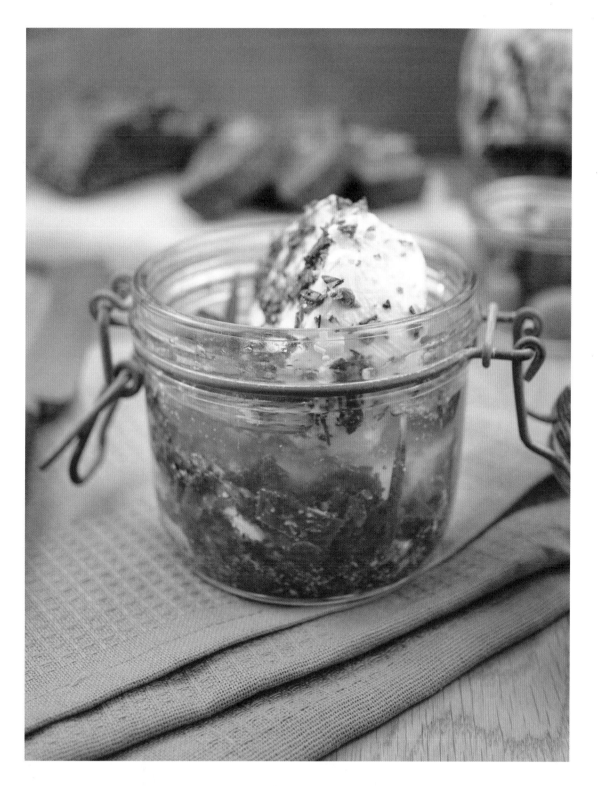

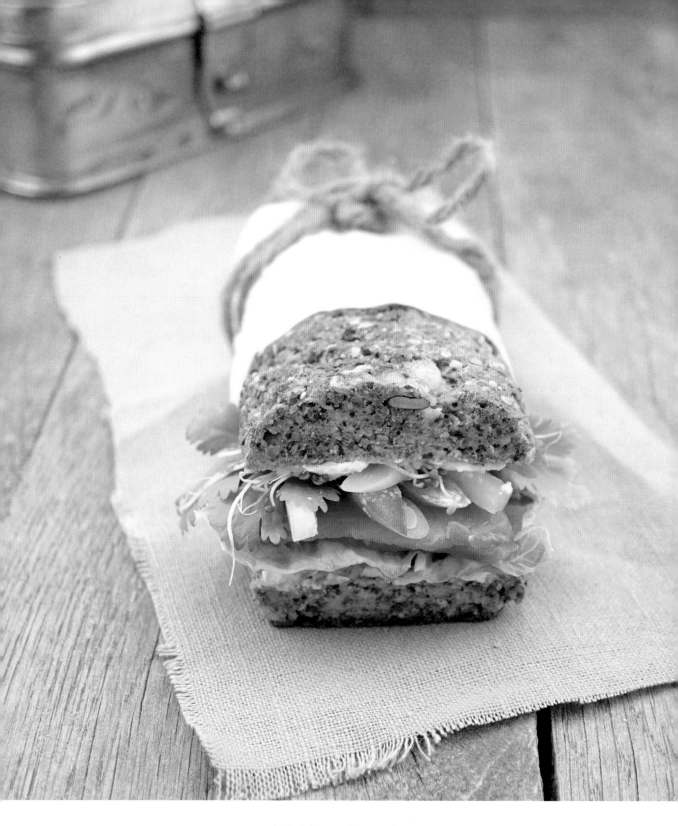

Cottage baguette
wholesome and vital

30g (1oz) ground almonds
25g (scant 1oz) ground
  hazelnuts
30g (1oz) psyllium husks
10g (¼oz) coconut flour
10g (¼oz) cream of tartar
3 eggs
125g (4½oz) cottage cheese
1 tbsp cider vinegar
½ tsp salt
pinch of ground coriander
30g (1oz) shelled hemp seeds
30g (1oz) chia seeds
15g (½oz) sunflower seeds
10g (¼oz) pumpkin seeds

Preheat the oven to 200°C (400°F/Gas 6). Line a baking tray with baking parchment.

Combine the almonds, hazelnuts, psyllium husks, coconut flour, and cream of tartar in a bowl. Whisk the eggs in a separate bowl and stir in the cottage cheese, cider vinegar, salt and coriander. Add the nut and flour mixture to the egg mixture and combine everything thoroughly.

Add the hemp, chia, sunflower, and pumpkin seeds to the dough mixture and stir them in. Lay the dough out lengthways on the baking parchment and shape it into a baguette.

Cut the surface of the dough several times with a knife. Bake the baguette in the centre of the oven for 30–40 minutes, until crisp and golden brown. Remove from the tray and leave to cool on a wire rack. Pack up a portion of the baguette in a container to take with you, leaving it plain or adding a topping, as desired.

OUR TIP — you can also make four delicious low-carb cottage rolls from this dough. Just shorten the cooking time to 25–30 minutes.

At home	At work	Serves	Kcal	Protein	Carbs	Fat
10 + 40 mins	0 min	4	305	18g	8g	20g

"Oopsies"
protein buns

3 eggs
100g (3½oz) full-fat
  cream cheese
salt

Preheat the oven to 200°C (400°C/Gas 6). Line 2 baking trays with baking parchment.

Separate the eggs. Beat the egg whites in a bowl using a hand-held whisk until they are stiff. In a separate bowl, stir together the cream cheese and egg yolks and season the mixture with a little salt. Fold the beaten egg whites carefully into this mixture using a balloon whisk or spatula.

Using a ladle, immediately scoop 4 dollops of the dough mixture onto each of the baking trays – making sure the blobs of dough aren't too close, otherwise the oopsies will merge together.

Bake the oopsies on the lower and central shelf of the oven for 15–20 minutes. Remove from the tray and leave to cool on a wire rack. Pack them up in a container to take with you, leaving them plain or adding a topping, as desired.

OUR TIP – oopsies can be filled with whatever topping you fancy and they also work well as burger buns.

At home	At work	Serves	Kcal	Protein	Carbs	Fat
10 + 20 mins	0 min	8	65	3g	1g	5g

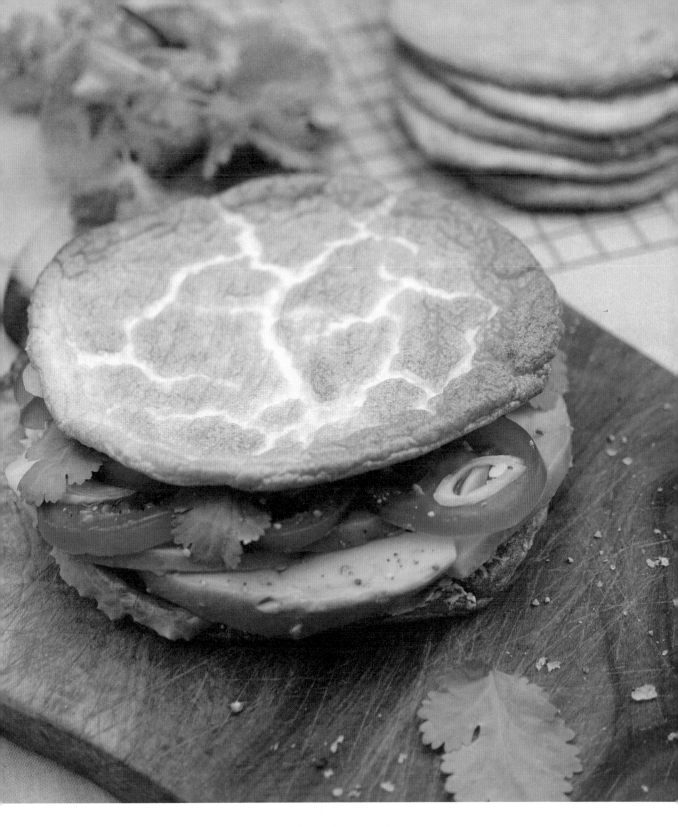

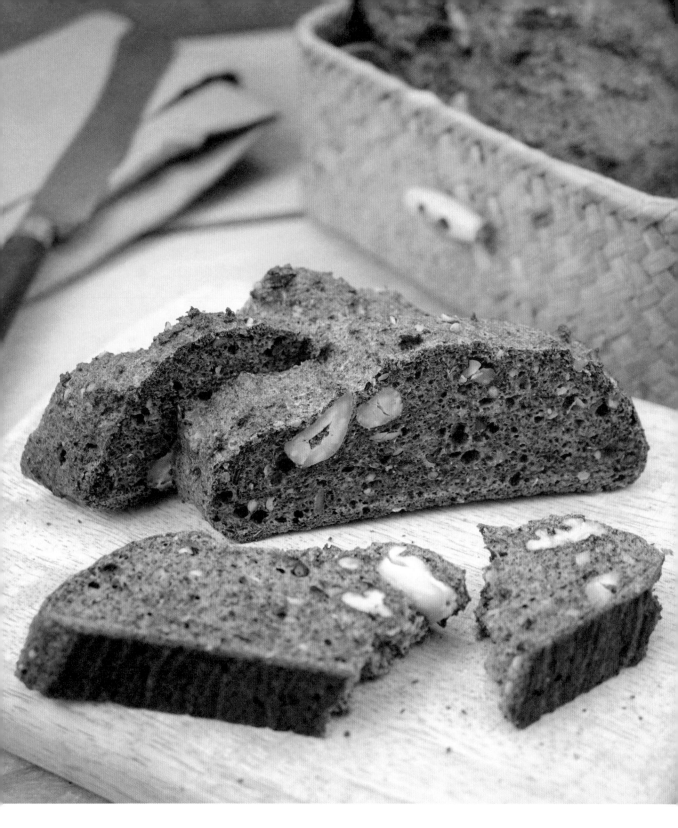

Nut bread
power loaf

4 eggs
175g (6oz) full-fat fromage frais
25g (scant 1oz) cashews
25g (scant 1oz) pecans
10g (¼oz) psyllium husks
½ tsp ground coriander
1 tsp salt
50g (1¾oz) hemp flour
30g (1oz) linseed flour
10g (¼oz) shelled hemp seeds
10g (¼oz) linseeds

Preheat the oven to 180°C (350°C/Gas 4). Line a baking tray with baking parchment.

Separate the eggs. Beat the egg whites in a bowl using a hand-held whisk until they are stiff. In a separate bowl, stir together the egg yolks and the fromage frais.

Roughly chop the cashews and pecans. Mix together the psyllium husks, coriander, salt, hemp and linseed flours, hemp seeds, and linseeds. Stir this mixture into the fromage frais mix. Add the cashews and pecans then carefully fold in the beaten egg whites. Finally, knead everything together to form a dough.

Allow the dough to rest for around 5 minutes, then shape it into a loaf on the baking parchment. Use a knife to make incisions in the top of the loaf then bake in the centre of the oven for 50–60 minutes. Remove the bread from the tray and leave to cool on a wire rack. Store in a container.

OUR TIP — a practical option for packed lunches is to make two smaller loaves from this dough. The baking time should then be shortened to 35–45 minutes.

At home	At work	Serves	Kcal	Protein	Carbs	Fat
15 + 60 mins	0 min	8	156	10g	3g	10g

Spelt and hemp bread

with sunflower seeds

7g sachet dried yeast (or
  ½ cube fresh yeast)
1 tbsp agave syrup
1 tbsp salt
250g (9oz) wholemeal
  spelt flour
225g (8oz) spelt flour with
  a high gluten content
25g (scant 1oz) linseed flour
3 tbsp sunflower seeds
2 tbsp linseeds
2 tbsp shelled hemp seeds
1 tbsp chia seeds

Dissolve the yeast in about 3½ tablespoons of lukewarm water and add the agave syrup. In a large bowl, combine the salt with all the different types of flour, the sunflower seeds, linseeds, hemp, and chia seeds.

Gradually add 250–300ml (9–10fl oz) lukewarm water to the yeast liquid, then knead everything together thoroughly for 5 to 10 minutes, until you have a stretchy dough. If the dough remains too sticky, knead in a bit of additional flour. Leave the dough covered in a warm place for around 1 hour to prove, until it has roughly doubled in size.

Preheat the oven to 220°C (425°F/Gas 7). Line a loaf tin with baking parchment. Knead the bread dough thoroughly once more, shape it into a loaf, and place it in the tin. Bake the bread in the centre of the oven for around 15 minutes, then lower the oven temperature to 160°C (325°F/Gas 3) and continue to cook the bread for an additional 15–20 minutes, until done.

Remove from the oven and leave the bread to cool in the tin for about 10 minutes, then release it from the tin and allow to cool down completely on a wire rack. Store in a container.

At home	At work	Serves	Kcal	Protein	Carbs	Fat
15 + 95 mins	0 min	16	130	6g	21g	2g

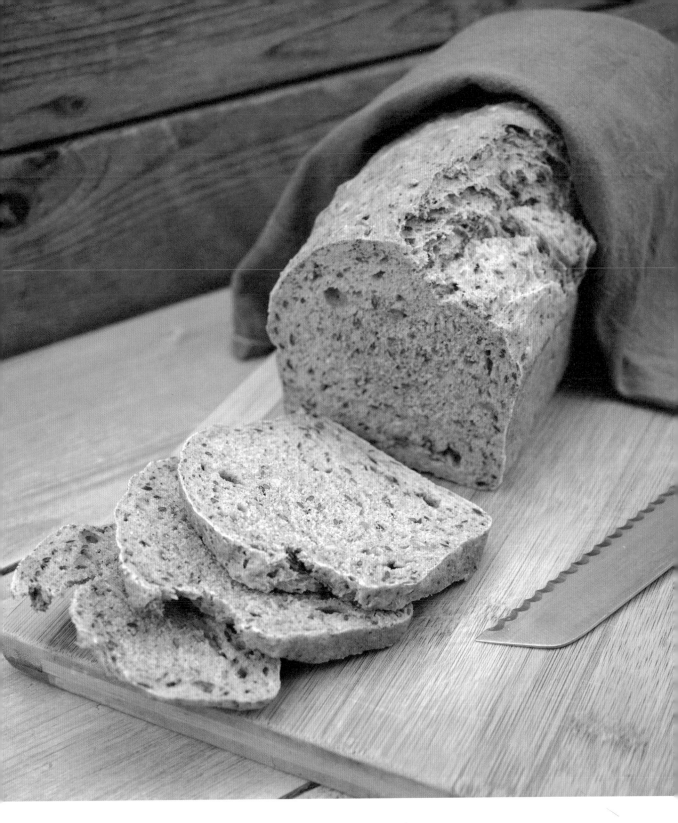

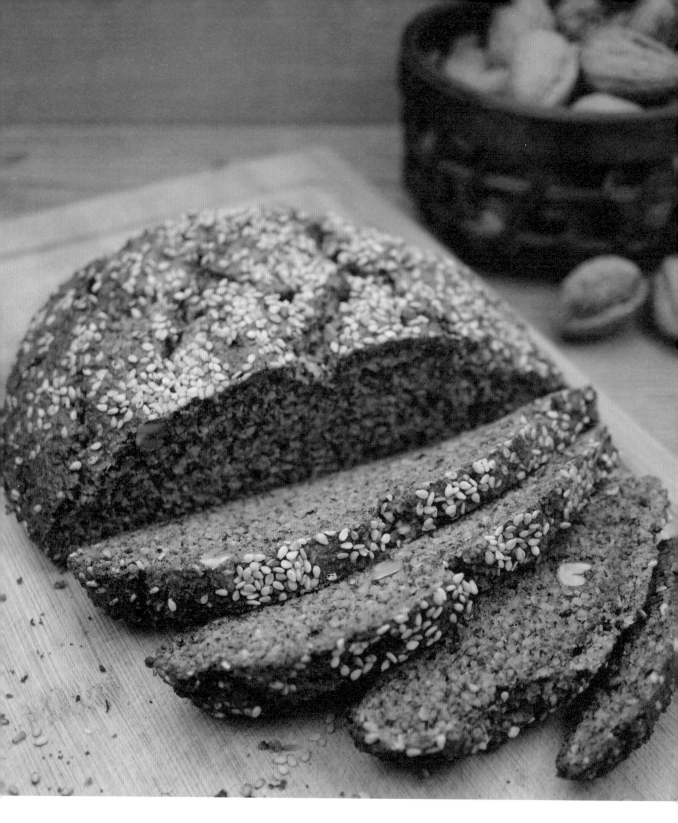

Walnut bread
with crunchy nuts

6 walnuts
30g (1oz) soft butter
2 eggs
3 tbsp yogurt
about 1 tsp agave syrup
pinch of salt
2 tbsp ground walnuts
200g (7oz) ground almonds
½ tsp bicarbonate of soda
2 tbsp white sesame seeds

Preheat the oven to 200°C (400°F/Gas 6). Line a baking tray with baking parchment.

Crack open the walnuts, remove the kernels from their shells, and chop roughly. Beat the butter in a bowl using a hand-held whisk until light and fluffy, then add the eggs and mix everything well. Stir the yogurt, agave syrup, and salt into the butter and egg mixture.

In a separate bowl, combine the ground walnuts, almonds, and bicarbonate of soda. Add this nut mixture to the egg mixture and stir everything together to form a dough. Finally, mix in the chopped walnuts.

Shape or press the dough to create a round loaf on the baking parchment. Scatter the loaf with sesame seeds and press these in slightly. Bake the walnut bread in the centre of the oven for 30 minutes, then lower the temperature to 180°C (350°F/Gas 4) and cook the bread for an additional 10–15 minutes, until done.

Remove the bread from the tray and leave to cool on a wire rack. Store in a container.

At home	At work	Serves	Kcal	Protein	Carbs	Fat
15 + 45 mins	0 min	10	200	8g	2g	17g

Buttermilk rolls
lovingly home-made

250g (9oz) buttermilk
½ cube of yeast (25g/scant 1oz)
350g (12oz) spelt flour with a
   high gluten content
1 tsp honey or a bit of
   low-calorie sweetener such
   as Stevia
1 tsp salt

In a saucepan, heat the buttermilk until lukewarm, then dissolve the yeast into it. Add the flour, honey, and salt and knead together to form a dough. Cover the dough and leave to prove in a warm place for around 30 minutes. Knead again and use some flour to help you shape 6 rolls from the mixture. Line a baking tray with baking parchment. Leave the rolls to prove on the tray for 15 minutes. Preheat the oven to 220°C (425°F/Gas 7). Bake the rolls in the centre of the oven for 15–20 minutes. Remove and leave to cool, then pack them in a container.

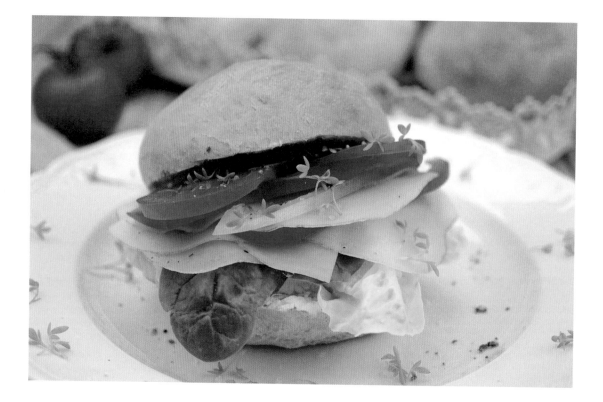

At home	At work	Serves	Kcal	Protein	Carbs	Fat
25 + 65 mins	0 min	6	220	9g	41g	1g

Low-carb rolls
with sunflower seeds

50g (1¾oz) linseed flour
15g (½oz) coconut flour
10g (¼oz) ground walnuts
15g (½oz) psyllium husks
1 tsp cream of tartar
1 tsp salt
1 tsp dried oregano
30g (1oz) sunflower seeds
5g (⅛oz) chia seeds
1 egg white

In a large bowl, combine all the ingredients except the egg white. Stir in 130ml (4½fl oz) boiling water with a fork, then knead everything by hand. Beat the egg white until stiff, add to the mixture, and knead everything together until you have a consistent dough. Line a baking tray with baking parchment. Shape the dough into 3 rolls; leave these to rest on the tray for 10 minutes. Preheat the oven to 180°C (350°F/Gas 4). Bake the rolls in the centre of the oven for around 30 minutes. Remove, allow to cool, then pack them up in a container to take with you.

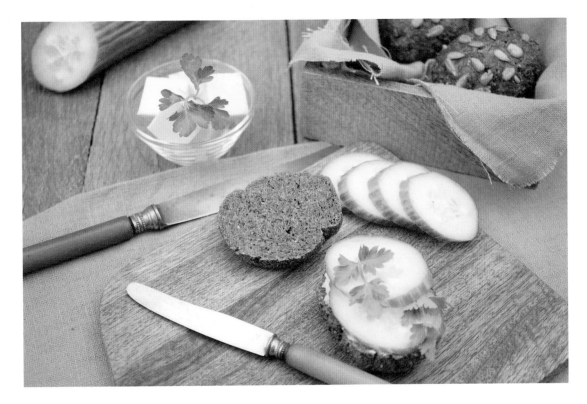

At home	At work	Serves	Kcal	Protein	Carbs	Fat
30 + 30 mins	0 min	3	180	11g	6g	8g

Fitness baguette

with a delicate hint of fennel, anise, and caraway

1 sachet fennel, anise, and
   caraway tea
30g (1oz) linseed flour
30g (1oz) ground almonds
40g (1¼oz) coconut flour
15g (½oz) psyllium husk powder
½ tsp salt
15g (½oz) cream of tartar
2 eggs
150g (5½oz) full-fat fromage frais
1 tsp cider vinegar

Place the tea bag in a mug, pour boiling hot water over it, and leave to steep for 10 minutes.

In a bowl, combine the linseed flour, almonds, coconut flour, and psyllium husks, then stir in the salt and cream of tartar. In a separate bowl, mix together the eggs, fromage frais, and vinegar. Add 1½ tablespoons of hot tea and the egg-fromage frais mix to the dry ingredients and knead everything together to form a dough.

Line a baking tray with baking parchment. Shape the dough into a loaf and place this on the baking parchment, making several diagonal incisions in the surface with a knife. Leave the dough to prove for 30 minutes.

Meanwhile, preheat the oven to 200°C (400°F/Gas 6). Bake the bread in the centre of the oven for 40–50 minutes, until golden brown. Remove from the tray and leave to cool on a wire rack. Store the baguette in a container until ready to use.

At home	At work	Serves	Kcal	Protein	Carbs	Fat
15 + 80 mins	0 min	4	191	14g	8g	9g

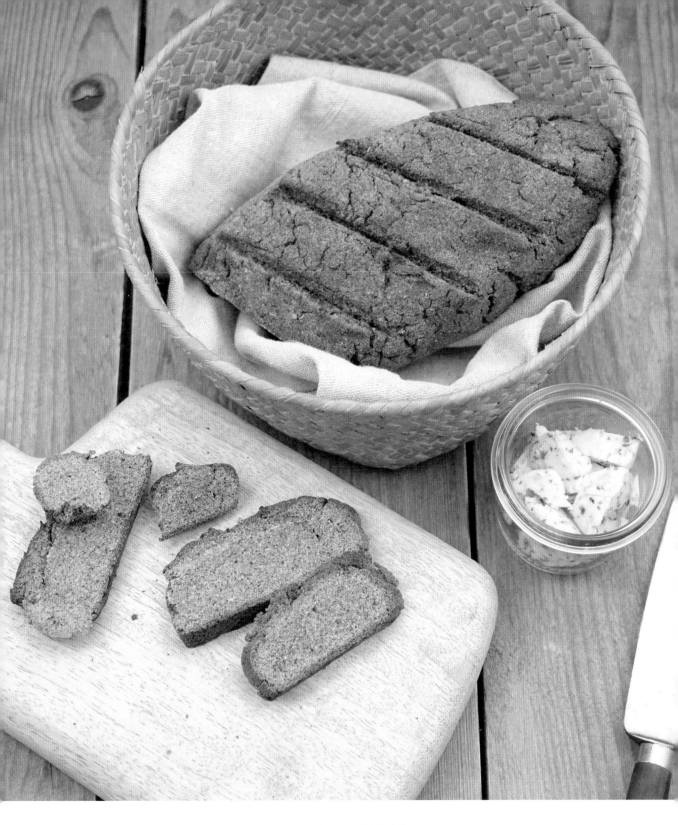

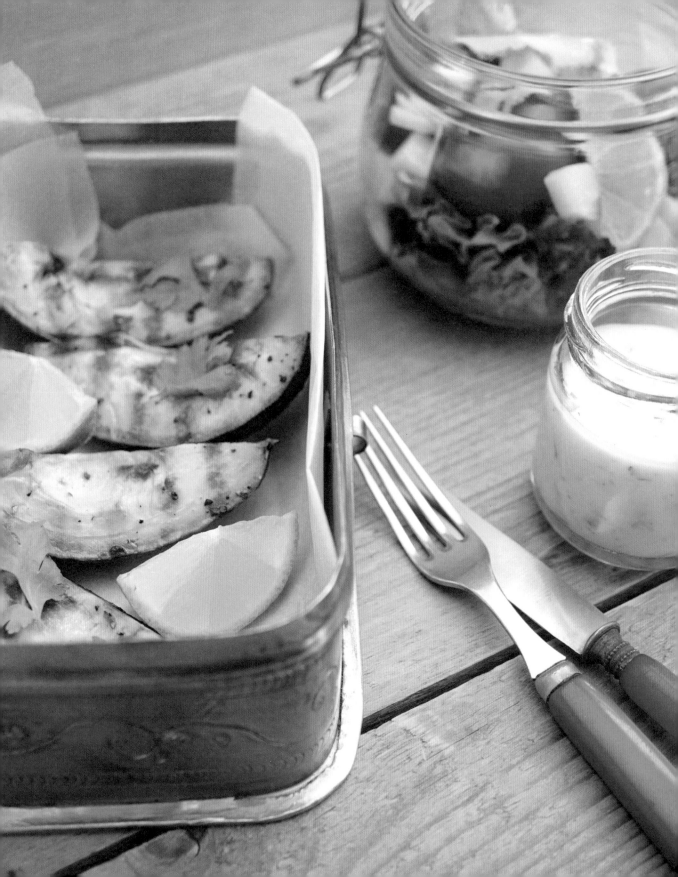

VEGETARIAN

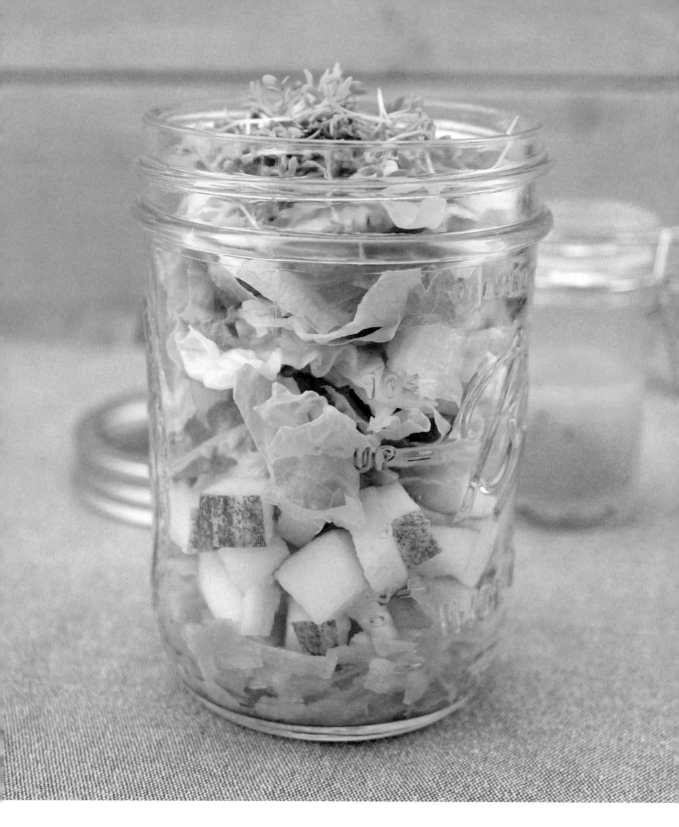

VEGETARIAN

Apple and carrot salad

with cress

FOR THE SALAD
1 carrot, finely grated
2 tsp lemon juice
1 tsp olive oil
1 small apple, cored and
    cut into bite-sized cubes
½ romaine lettuce,
    roughly chopped
1 tbsp cress leaves

FOR THE DRESSING
3 tbsp olive oil
2 tbsp lemon juice
1 tbsp orange juice
1 tsp cress leaves
salt and freshly ground
    black pepper

Drizzle the carrot with about 1 tsp lemon juice and the olive oil. Drizzle the diced apple with the remaining lemon juice.

Layer up the grated carrot, apple, and lettuce in a tall jar and finish off with the cress leaves. Close the jar.

To make the dressing, put all the ingredients into a small jar. Seal the jar and shake vigorously so the ingredients combine to form a homogenous dressing. Store the salad and dressing in the fridge until ready to serve.

AT WORK — shake the dressing again in the closed jar, then add to the salad.

At home	At work	Serves	Kcal	Protein	Carbs	Fat
10 mins	1 min	1	380	2g	17g	32g

Carrot and cucumber noodles
with lime dressing

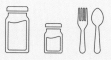

FOR THE SALAD

1 carrot

½ cucumber, peeled

1 tbsp white sesame seeds

½ romaine lettuce, cut into
  thin strips

1 spring onion, root discarded,
  white thinly sliced

¼ red chilli, deseeded and
  thinly sliced

salt and freshly ground
  black pepper

FOR THE DRESSING

juice of ½ lime

2 ½ tbsp olive oil

1 tbsp sesame oil

1 tsp agave syrup

½ tsp salt

Use a spiralizer to cut the carrot and cucumber into long vegetable noodles. Toast the sesame seeds in a dry pan until they release their aroma.

Combine all the prepared salad ingredients carefully in a salad bowl. Season the salad with salt and pepper, transfer to a tall jar, and close.

For the dressing, place all the ingredients in a bowl and mix thoroughly. Pour the dressing into a small jar and close. Store the salad and dressing in the fridge until ready to serve.

AT WORK — add the dressing to the salad, close the jar, and shake. Eat the salad straight from the jar or tip it out onto a plate.

At home	At work	Serves	Kcal	Protein	Carbs	Fat
10 mins	1 min	1	169	4g	15g	11g

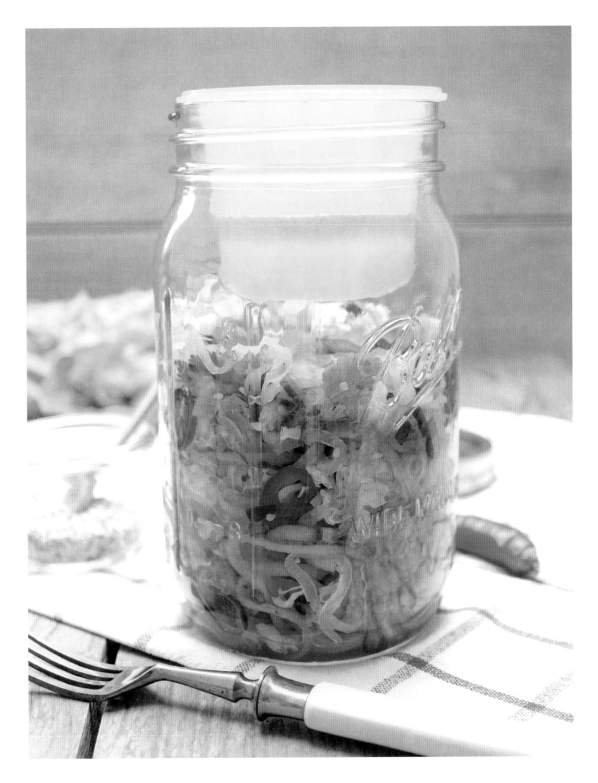

VEGETARIAN

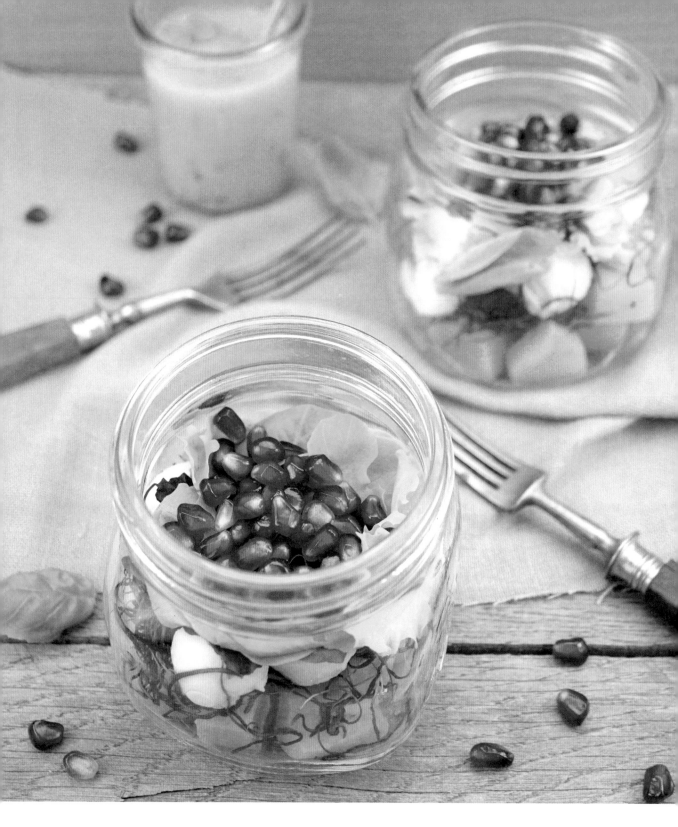

Squash salad

with a basil and squash dressing

300g (10oz) butternut squash,
    peeled, deseeded, and cut
    into small cubes
slice of ginger, peeled
2 sprigs of basil leaves
1 tsp groundnut oil
salt and freshly ground
    black pepper
2 tbsp beetroot shoots
10 mini mozzarella balls
2–3 round lettuce leaves,
    roughly chopped
2 tbsp pomegranate seeds

Preheat the oven to 180°C (350°F/Gas 4). Line a baking tray with baking parchment. Spread the squash over the baking parchment and roast in the centre of the oven for around 15 minutes, until soft but not mushy. Remove the squash from the oven and leave to cool.

To make the dressing, put around 60g (2oz) of the cooked squash into a blender beaker. Add the ginger, basil, groundnut oil, and 75ml (2½fl oz) water to the squash and use a hand-held blender to process thoroughly. Season the dressing with salt and pepper to taste and pour into a small jar. Close the jar and keep the dressing in the fridge until ready to use.

To make the salad, divide the remaining squash between 2 jars. Rinse the shoots briefly in cold water in a sieve, leave to drain then add to the squash. Lay the mozzarella balls on top. Add the lettuce leaves on top of the mozzarella balls and finish off with the pomegranate seeds. Close the jars and store the salad in the fridge until ready to serve.

AT WORK — tip the salad out onto a plate and drizzle over the dressing using a spoon. Or pour the dressing over the salad in the jar and eat straight from the container.

At home	At work	Serves	Kcal	Protein	Carbs	Fat
30 mins	1 min	2	185	8g	18g	9g

Multi-coloured salad
with quinoa

FOR THE SALAD

1 tsp pine nuts

30g (1oz) quinoa

1 tsp orange juice

salt and freshly ground
   black pepper

7 cherry tomatoes, halved

60g (2oz) orange pepper,
   deseeded and finely chopped

40g (1¼oz) yellow pepper,
   deseeded and finely chopped

1 red cabbage leaf, about
   20g (¾oz), thinly sliced

1 round lettuce leaf, finely
   chopped

FOR THE DRESSING

2 tbsp orange juice

1 tbsp lemon juice

1–2 tsp agave syrup (to taste)

Toast the pine nuts in a dry pan until golden brown, remove from the pan, and leave to cool.

Wash the quinoa thoroughly in a sieve under running water. Transfer the quinoa to a pan, cover with water, and simmer uncovered for 8–10 minutes, until cooked. Drain the water, stir the orange juice into the quinoa, and leave to soak briefly. Season the orange quinoa with salt and pepper to taste and leave to cool.

To make the dressing, stir together the orange and lemon juice. Sweeten the dressing to taste with some agave syrup, then pour into a small jar and seal. Store the dressing in the fridge until ready to use.

Transfer the quinoa to a jar then arrange layers of tomatoes, pepper pieces, cabbage, and lettuce one after the other, finishing off with a scattering of pine nuts. Close the jar and keep the salad in the fridge until you are ready to serve.

AT WORK — add the dressing to the salad and eat straight from the jar, or serve on a plate.

At home	At work	Serves	Kcal	Protein	Carbs	Fat
15 mins	1 min	1	170	5g	23g	5g

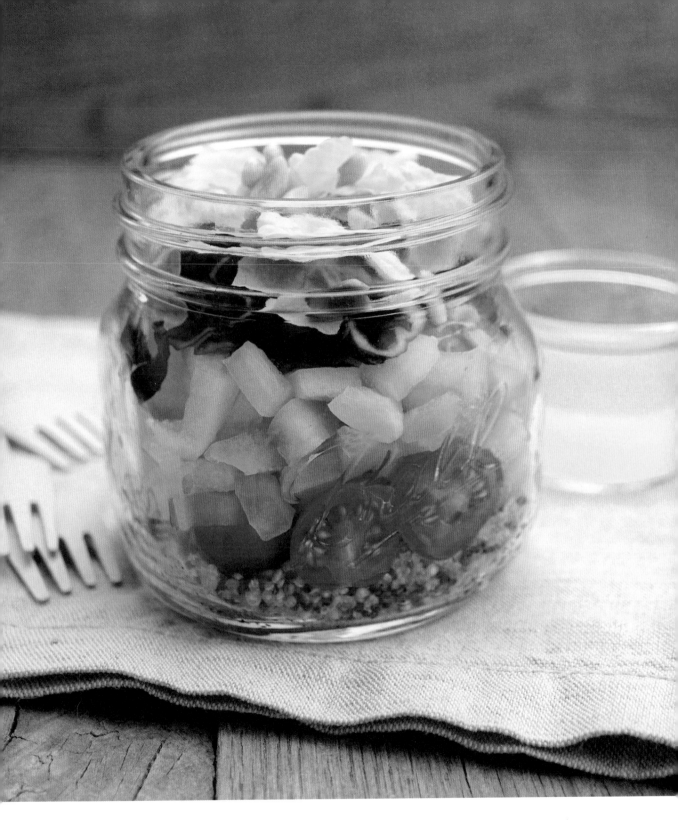

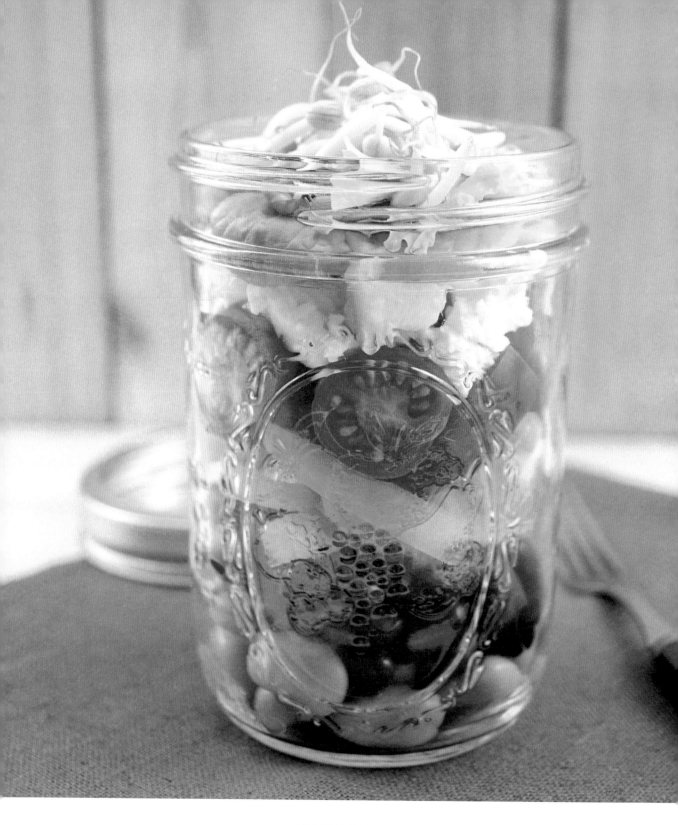

Pepper and bean salad

with feta

50g (1¾oz) tinned haricot
    or cannellini beans
50g (1¾oz) tinned kidney beans
small piece of orange pepper,
    about 25g (scant 1 oz),
    deseeded and sliced
    into strips
small piece of red pepper,
    about 25g (scant 1 oz),
    deseeded and sliced
    into strips
2 yellow cherry tomatoes,
    halved
1 red cherry tomato, halved
30g (1oz) feta
handful of mixed lettuce leaves,
    roughly chopped
1 tbsp bean sprouts
salt and freshly ground black
    pepper (in lidded dispensers)

Rinse the haricot or cannellini beans and the kidney beans thoroughly in a sieve under running water and leave to drain. Transfer all the beans to a jar.

Layer the pepper strips on top of the beans. Add the tomatoes to the jar. Crumble the feta with your fingers and scatter over the tomatoes, then add the lettuce to the jar.

Blanche the bean sprouts in boiling water for about 5 seconds, rinse under cold water in a sieve, and leave to drain. Scatter the bean sprouts over the salad. Close the jar and store the salad in the fridge until ready to serve.

AT WORK — tip the salad out onto a plate and season with salt and pepper. Alternatively, eat the salad straight from the jar.

At home	At work	Serves	Kcal	Protein	Carbs	Fat
10 mins	1 min	1	190	14g	14g	7g

Tomato salad with cottage cheese
and basil

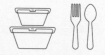

200g (7oz) cottage cheese
salt and freshly ground
    black pepper
zest and juice of 1 organic
    lemon
2 sprigs of basil leaves
1 tsp olive oil
5 red cherry tomatoes, halved
5 yellow cherry tomatoes,
  . halved
3 radishes, thinly sliced

Season the cottage cheese with salt and pepper and stir in the lemon zest.

Using a pestle and mortar, grind the basil leaves with the olive oil, pepper, and 1–2 tablespoons of lemon juice to create the dressing. Transfer the dressing to a bowl and toss the tomatoes and radishes into it.

Pack up the cottage cheese and tomato salad in 2 separate containers and close. Store both in the fridge until ready to serve.

AT WORK — add the tomato salad to the cottage cheese and eat straight from the container. Or arrange the cheese and salad together on a plate.

At home	At work	Serves	Kcal	Protein	Carbs	Fat
10 mins	1 min	1	270	26g	9g	14g

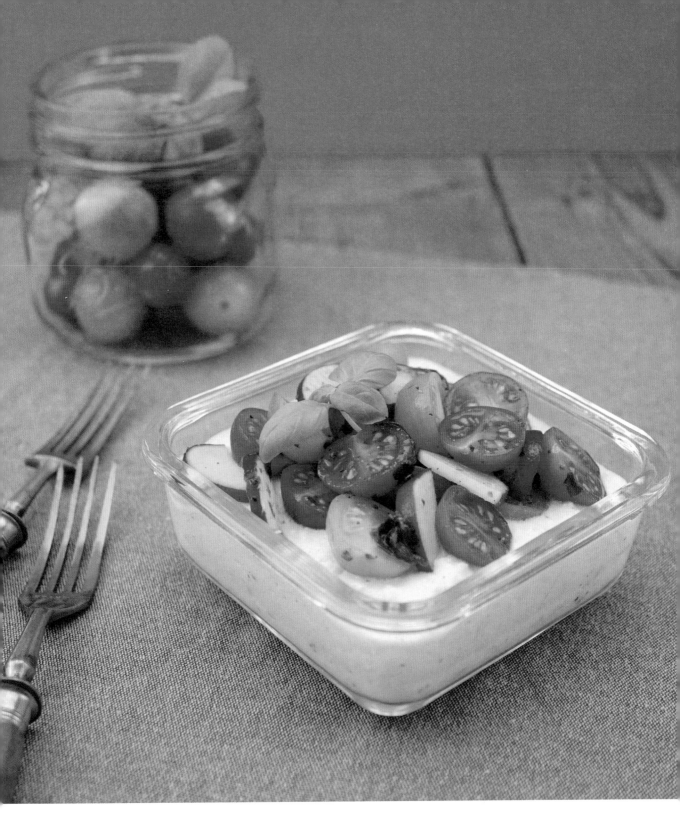

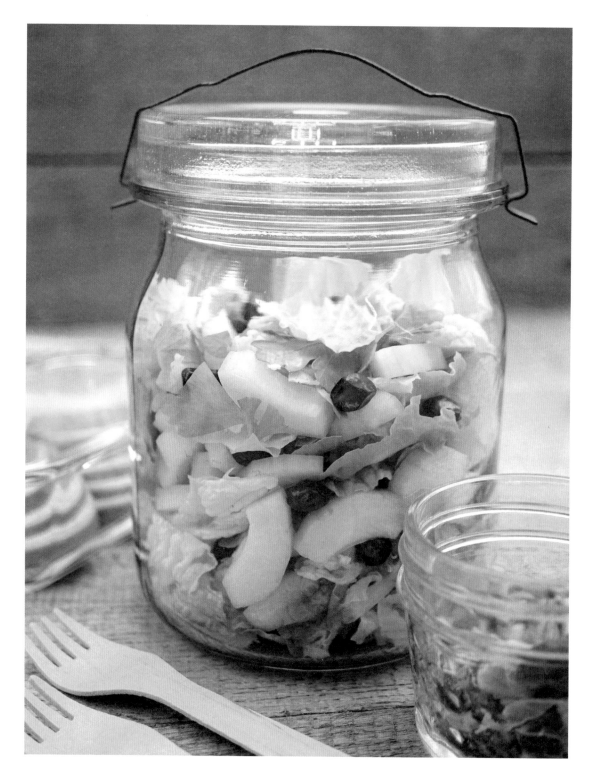

VEGETARIAN

Cucumber power
with avocado

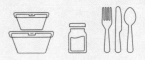

½ cucumber, sliced lengthways, deseeded, and chopped into small pieces

2 handfuls of green salad, roughly chopped

1–2 sprigs of coriander leaves

1 tbsp pomegranate seeds

1 avocado, pitted, flesh removed and sliced

juice of ½ lime

2 tbsp mixed nuts

1 tbsp white sesame seeds

salt and freshly ground pepper (in lidded dispensers)

Place the cucumber, salad, and coriander in a container. Add the pomegranate seeds.

Drizzle the avocado slices with lime juice to prevent them from going brown. Pack the avocado slices into a separate container. Put the mixed nuts and sesame seeds into another container. Close all your containers and store the salad mixture and the avocado in the fridge until ready to serve.

AT WORK — arrange your cucumber power salad on 2 plates and season with salt and pepper. Add the avocado and the nut mixture. The salad can be drizzled with some lime juice or olive oil or with a salad dressing (for example, from the Apple and carrot salad, see p83, or from the Carrot and cucumber noodles, see p84).

At home	At work	Serves	Kcal	Protein	Carbs	Fat
10 mins	2 mins	2	330	6g	5g	32g

Kimchi

spicy Korean Chinese cabbage

300g (10oz) Chinese cabbage,
   tough stems removed and
   leaves roughly chopped
½ carrot, cut into batons
½ spring onion, root discarded,
   white thinly sliced
2 tbsp salt
2 garlic cloves, crushed
2 tbsp soy sauce
2 tbsp chilli flakes

Place the cabbage, carrot, and spring onion in a bowl, sprinkle with the salt, and leave to steep for 30 minutes. Transfer the vegetables to a sieve then rinse them off thoroughly under cold water and leave to drain. Then use your hands to squeeze any excess water from the vegetables and transfer to a large bowl.

Put the garlic in a small bowl. Add the soy sauce and chilli flakes and stir. Add this mixture to the cabbage and combine everything thoroughly with your hands, working the ingredients for several minutes.

Either eat the kimchi straight away, or transfer it to a sterile, dry jar with a sealed lid and leave to mature in the fridge. Fill the jar only three-quarters full with kimchi to leave room for it to mature. The kimchi will gradually collapse down in the jar. The longer the kimchi is left to infuse in the fridge, the more aromatic its flavour becomes. Kimchi can be kept refrigerated for at least 2 weeks, and often much longer.

OUR TIP — if you fancy experimenting with kimchi a bit, add a sweet element, perhaps in the form of some puréed apple or pear.

At home	At work	Serves	Kcal	Protein	Carbs	Fat
45 mins	0 min	4	40	2g	5g	1g

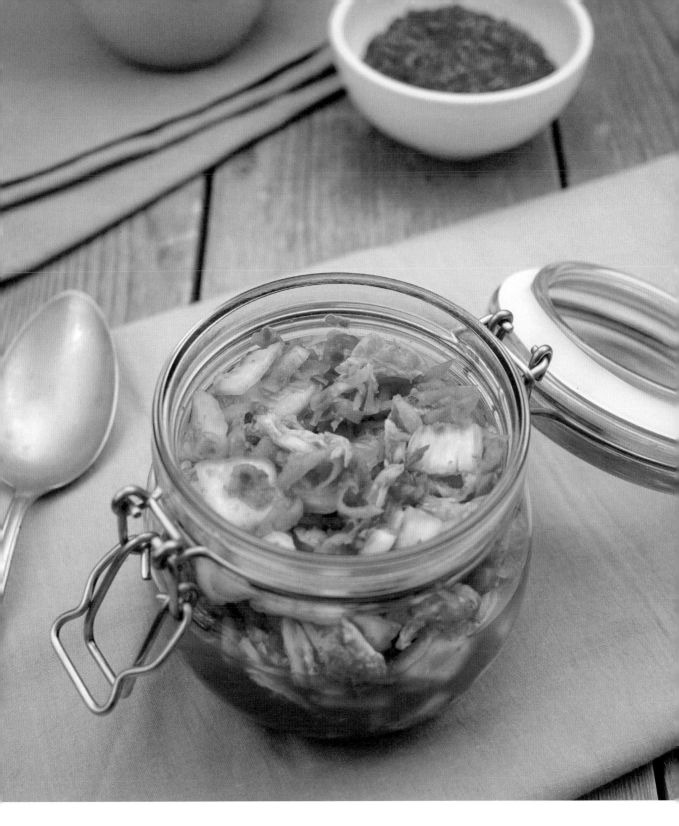

VEGETARIAN

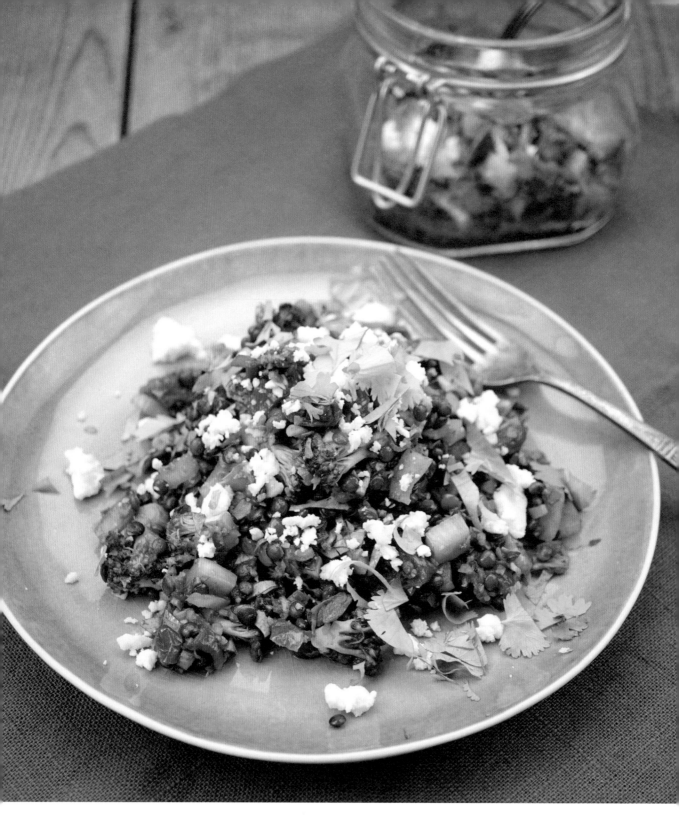

Beluga lentil salad
with feta

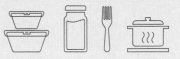

50g (1¾oz) beluga lentils
1 tbsp coconut oil
1 shallot, finely diced
2 tsp tomato purée
1 tbsp cider vinegar
60g (2oz) broccoli florets
60g (2oz) fennel, thinly sliced
1 spring onion, root discarded
    and white finely sliced
grated zest of 1 organic lemon
3 tbsp soy sauce
pinch of ground star anise
pinch of ground cumin
salt and freshly ground
    black pepper
1 tsp goji berries
1 pecan nut
1 small sundried tomato
30g (1oz) feta
2 sprigs of coriander

Cover the beluga lentils with water in a bowl and leave to soak for 12 hours, ideally overnight. Drain the lentils in a sieve and rinse with water.

Heat the coconut oil in a small pan and sauté the shallots. Add the lentils plus the tomato purée and stir everything together. Deglaze with the cider vinegar and 3½ tablespoons of water and leave to simmer for 15 minutes. Add the broccoli, fennel, and spring onion and top up with 60—100ml (2—3½fl oz) water. Simmer for a further 10 minutes, until the lentils are just cooked.

Stir the lemon zest, soy sauce, star anise, cumin, and some salt and pepper into the lentils. Finely chop the goji berries, pecans, and dried tomato and stir these in, too. Remove the pan from the heat and leave the lentil salad to cool down. Transfer to a jar and seal. Pack the feta and coriander in a separate container and store this in the fridge with the salad until ready to serve.

AT WORK — if desired, heat the salad in a pan. Crumble the feta over the salad with your fingers. Wash and dab dry the coriander, pluck off the leaves, chop coarsely, and add to the salad.

At home	At work	Serves	Kcal	Protein	Carbs	Fat
20 mins + 12 hrs	5 mins	2	225	12g	17g	11g

Red lentil salad
with harissa dressing

FOR THE SALAD
1 tbsp olive oil
1 shallot, diced
70g (2¼oz) red lentils
1–2cm piece of ginger, grated
1 garlic clove, diced
200ml (7fl oz) vegetable stock
45g (1½oz) courgette, cut
    into cubes
50g (1¾oz) red pepper,
    deseeded and cut into cubes
sprig of rosemary leaves,
    finely chopped
salt and freshly ground
    black pepper
45g (1½oz) spinach leaves,
    roughly chopped

FOR THE DRESSING
3 tbsp yogurt
½ tsp harissa paste
1 tsp lemon juice

FOR THE TOPPING
sprig of mint
sprig of flat-leaf parsley
15g (½oz) dried mixed berries
slice of lemon (optional)

Heat the olive oil in a small pan and sauté the shallot. Add the lentils, ginger, and garlic. Pour in the stock and simmer everything uncovered for around 15 minutes, until the lentils are just cooked.

Add the courgette and pepper to the lentils and warm gently, if necessary adding a bit more water. Add the rosemary and season to taste with salt and pepper. Remove the lentils from the pan and leave to cool before decanting into a container. Pack the spinach leaves in a separate container.

To make the dressing, stir together the yogurt, harissa, and lemon juice, plus some salt and pepper. Pour the dressing into a jar and seal. Pack the topping ingredients in a separate container. Store the salad, dressing, and topping ingredients in the fridge until ready to serve.

AT WORK — arrange the spinach on 2 plates and tip the lentils on top. If prefered, you can gently heat the lentil mixture beforehand. For the topping, pluck off the mint and parsley leaves, cut into strips, then add to the salad with the mixed berries, drizzling over a dash of lemon juice, if desired. Add the dressing to the salad.

At home	At work	Serves	Kcal	Protein	Carbs	Fat
30 mins	5 mins	2	195	9g	23g	7g

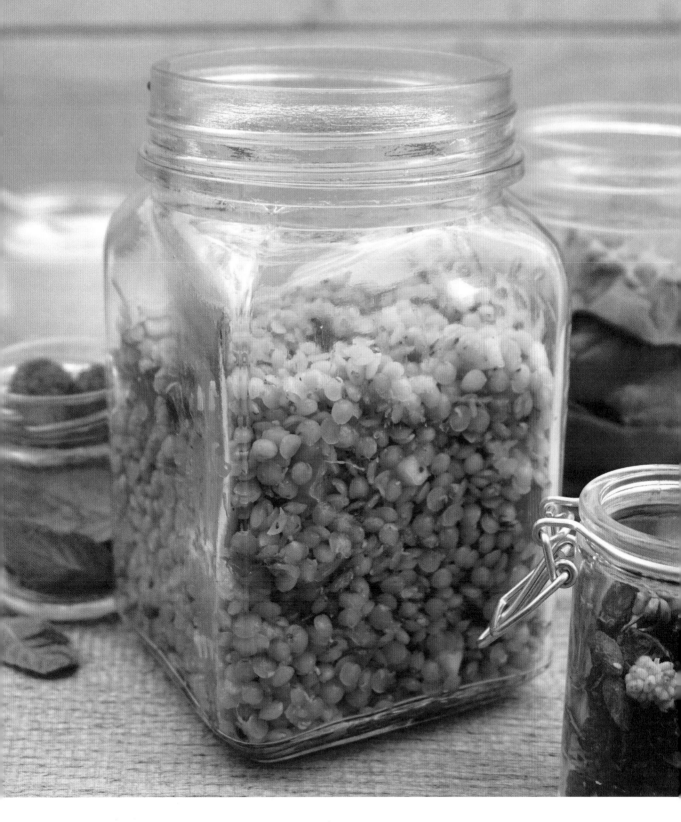

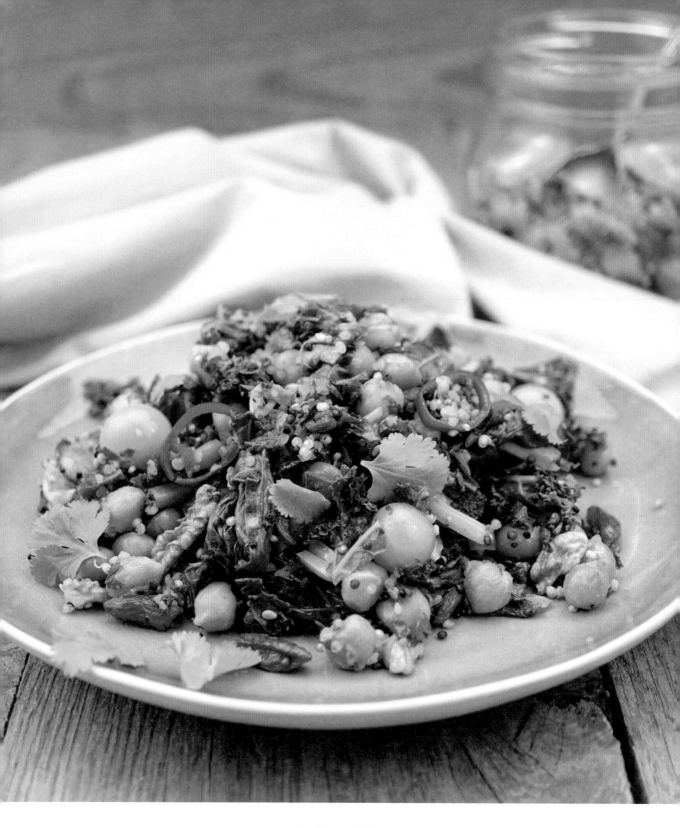

Kale and spinach salad
with an orange dressing

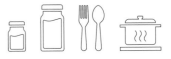

FOR THE SALAD
20g (¾oz) quinoa
50g (1¾oz) kale, stems removed
   and leaves chopped
40g (1¼oz) spinach, stalks
   removed and leaves chopped
50g (1¾oz) tinned chickpeas
1 garlic clove, finely chopped
¼ red chilli, deseeded and
   sliced into thin rings
20g (¾oz) walnuts, shelled and
   coarsely chopped
6 cape gooseberries (physalis
   fruit), leaves removed
1 tbsp butter
1 tsp goji berries, about 5g
sprig of coriander leaves

FOR THE DRESSING
2 tbsp orange juice
2 tbsp lemon juice
1 tsp agave syrup
salt

For the salad, wash the quinoa thoroughly in a sieve under running water. Cover with water in a small pan and simmer, uncovered, for 5–8 minutes, until just cooked. Rinse the chickpeas thoroughly in a sieve and leave to drain.

To make the dressing, stir together the orange juice, lemon juice, and agave syrup. Season the dressing to taste with salt. Drain the cooked quinoa in a sieve. Heat the butter in a large pan and sauté the kale until it wilts. Add the garlic and 1 tablespoon dressing and allow to cook briefly. Stir in the chickpeas and continue to cook everything for about another 5 minutes. Stir in the quinoa, chilli, walnuts, goji berries, cape gooseberries, and spinach and fry everything for 5 minutes. Add the coriander leaves to the salad.

Transfer the salad from the pan into a jar and leave to cool. Pour any remaining dressing into a small jar. Close both jars and store in the fridge.

AT WORK — the salad can be eaten cold or warmed up slightly, as you prefer.

At home	At work	Serves	Kcal	Protein	Carbs	Fat
20 mins	5 mins	1	465	10g	28g	22g

Pepper boats

with cream cheese

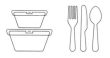

150g (5½oz) full-fat cream cheese
1 small tomato, seeds removed
    and flesh finely chopped
½ carrot, finely grated
1–2 cm piece of ginger, finely
    grated
juice of ½ lime
2–3 sprigs of chopped flat-leaf
    parsley leaves, plus extra to
    garnish (optional)
salt and freshly ground
    black pepper
6–8 colourful mini peppers,
    deseeded and halved
    lengthways

Combine the cream cheese with the diced tomato, grated carrot, and ginger, plus the lime juice in a bowl, mixing everything thoroughly. Add the parsley to the cream cheese mixture, season with salt and pepper, and stir.

Pack the pepper halves and the cream cheese mixture in separate containers and seal. Store both in the fridge until ready to serve.

AT WORK — arrange the pepper halves on two plates skin-side down. Fill the pepper halves with the cream cheese mixture and, if desired, scatter over some additional parsley.

At home	At work	Serves	Kcal	Protein	Carbs	Fat
15 mins	2 mins	2	230	7g	8g	19g

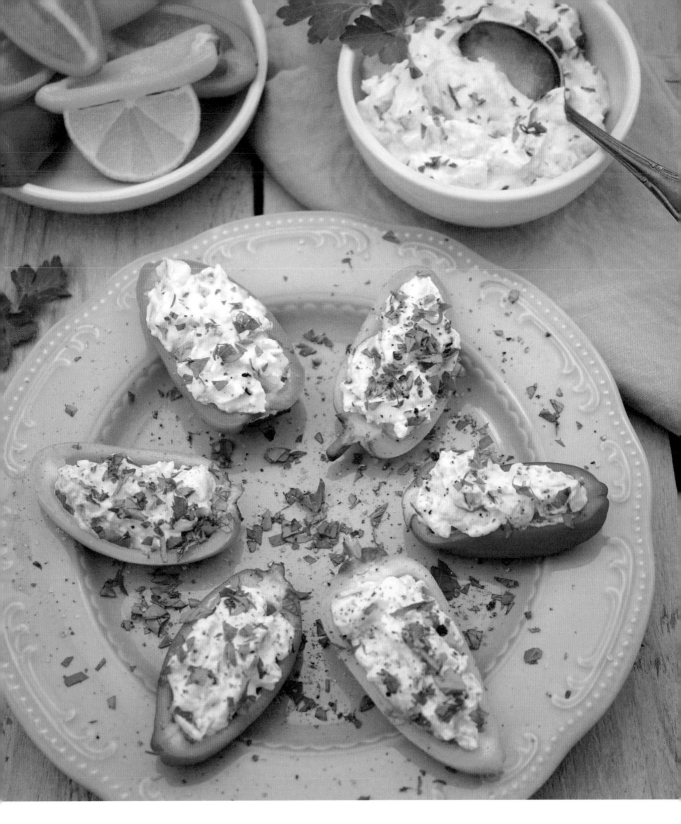

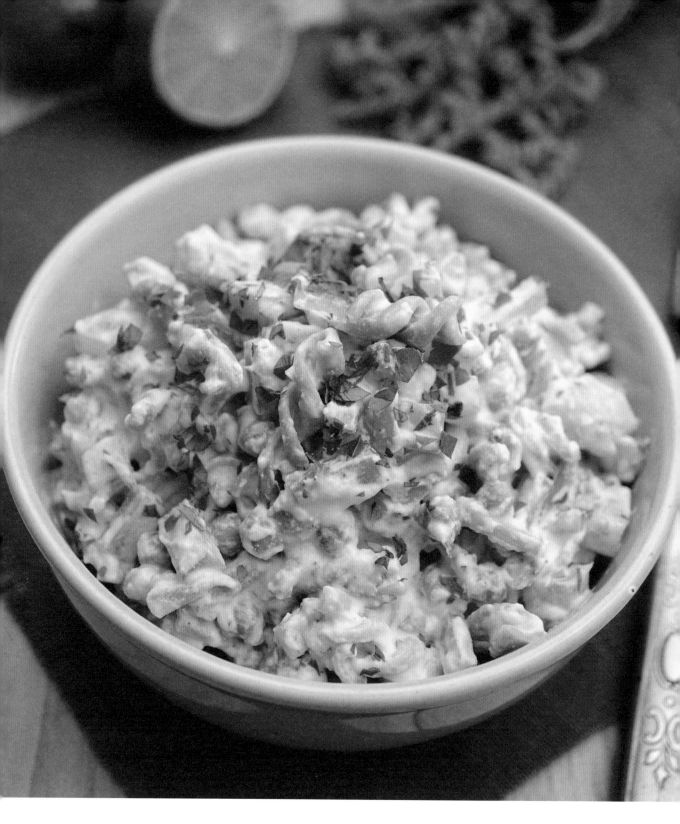

Chickpea pasta salad

with mixed vegetables

50g (1¾oz) chickpea pasta
   (such as chickpea fusilli from
   a health-food shop)
salt and freshly ground
   black pepper
40g (1¼oz) carrots, cut into
   small pieces
50g (1¾oz) peas (freshly
   podded or defrosted)
50g (1¾oz) yellow pepper,
   deseeded and cut into cubes
160g (5¾oz) yogurt
grated zest 1 organic lime
3 sprigs of flat-leaf parsley
   leaves, chopped

Cook the chickpea pasta in a large pan of salted boiling water for 3 minutes, then add the carrots and peas and continue to simmer for about 3 minutes. Drain the pasta and vegetables in a sieve, rinse in cold water, and leave to drain.

Mix the pasta and all the vegetables with the yogurt, lime zest, and parsley in a bowl. Season the salad to taste with salt and pepper, transfer to a container, and seal. Store the salad in the fridge until ready to serve.

OUR TIP — the ingredients in this pasta salad can be varied and substituted to create endless different options. For example, it also tastes fantastic with dried tomatoes and rocket or try adding some strips of roasted chicken breast and pieces of pineapple.

At home	At work	Serves	Kcal	Protein	Carbs	Fat
20 mins	0 min	1	225	16g	26g	6g

Courgette pasta salad

with toasted pine nuts

1 tbsp walnuts, roughly chopped

1 tbsp pine nuts

1 small courgette

1 tbsp lemon juice

1 tsp linseed

salt and freshly ground black pepper

50g (1¾oz) yellow pepper, deseeded and cut into small cubes

50g (1¾oz) orange pepper, deseeded and cut into small cubes

6 cherry tomatoes, halved

Toast the walnuts in a dry pan along with the pine nuts.

Use a spiralizer to turn the courgette into long, thin noodles. Toss the courgette noodles in a bowl with the lemon juice, walnuts, pine nuts, and linseed. Season the mixture with salt and pepper.

Transfer the courgette noodles into a jar. Then layer up the pepper pieces and tomatoes on top. Close the jar and store the salad in the fridge until ready to serve.

OUR TIP — the courgette salad can also be heated in a pan and eaten warm. To reheat, simply add 1 tablespoon olive oil to the salad in the pan.

At home	At work	Serves	Kcal	Protein	Carbs	Fat
10 mins	0 min	1	180	7g	13g	11g

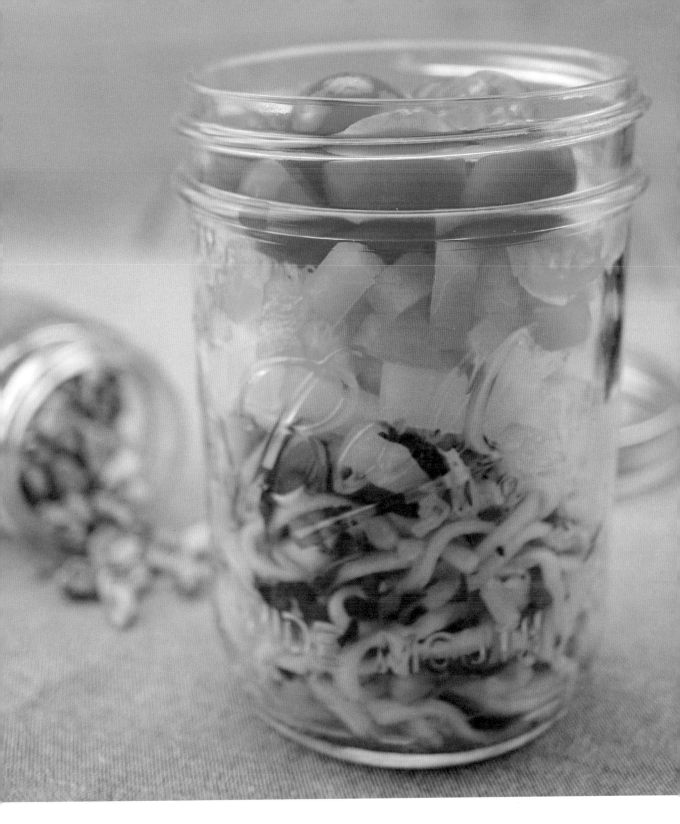

VEGETARIAN

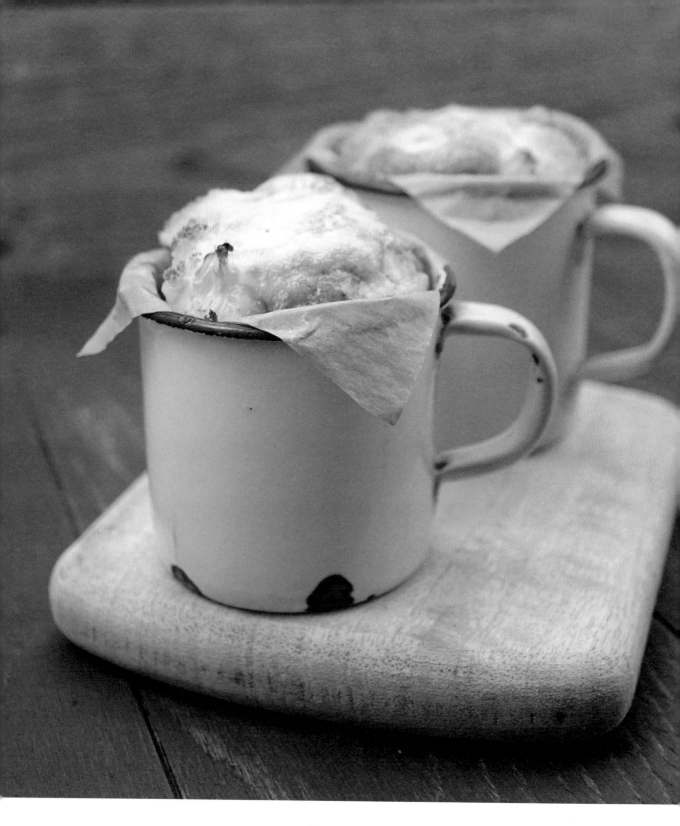

Cauliflower egg muffin

in a mug

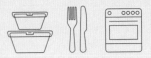

6 eggs
salt and freshly ground
  black pepper
200g (7oz) cauliflower florets

Preheat the oven to 240°C (475°F/Gas 9). Line 2 ovenproof mugs with baking parchment.

Whisk the eggs, then season with salt and pepper. Put the cauliflower florets into the mugs, pour over the eggs, and bake in the centre of the oven for 30 minutes.

Remove the mugs from the oven and leave the muffins to cool. Pack the muffins, still in their mugs, in a container and seal. Store the muffins in the fridge until ready to serve.

AT WORK — preheat the oven to 220°C (425°F/Gas 7). Heat the cauliflower and egg muffins in their mugs in the oven for 15 minutes. The muffins can also be reheated in the microwave, just be sure your mug is microwave safe. Heat the muffins all the way through.

OUR TIP — this recipe is also ideal as a quick "emergency fix" — just take eggs and your choice of vegetable to work and prepare on the spot. It tastes great with spinach, peppers, or mushrooms.

At home	At work	Serves	Kcal	Protein	Carbs	Fat
10 + 30 mins	15 mins	2	275	22g	5g	16g

Omelette rolls

with cream cheese filling

280g (9½oz) full-fat cream cheese
½ carrot, finely grated
1 tomato, finely diced
2 mini peppers, deseeded,
    1 pepper cut into cubes and
    1 pepper sliced into rings
½ red chilli, deseeded and
    finely chopped
juice of 1 lime
1–2 cm piece ginger, finely
    chopped
10g (¼oz) parmesan
salt and freshly ground
    black pepper
4 eggs
1 tsp olive oil

Mix the cream cheese with the carrot, tomato, diced pepper, chilli, and lime juice. Add the ginger and grate in the parmesan. Season the cream cheese mixture with salt and pepper and stir everything together once more.

Whisk the eggs in a bowl and season with salt and pepper. Heat half the olive oil in a pan and pour in half the egg mixture so that the base of the pan is covered. Let the omelette firm up briefly over a moderate heat, then turn it to finish cooking. Transfer the omelette from the pan onto a chopping board. Make a second omelette in the same way from the remaining egg mixture and transfer this to the chopping board, too.

Spread the omelettes with the cream cheese mixture, roll them up, transfer to a container, then seal. Pack the pepper rings in a separate container. Store the omelettes and pepper rings in the fridge until ready to serve.

AT WORK — lay the omelettes on a plate and serve with the pepper rings. If you wish, garnish with some lettuce, tomatoes, and herb leaves.

At home	At work	Serves	Kcal	Protein	Carbs	Fat
25 mins	1 min	2	595	26g	13g	49g

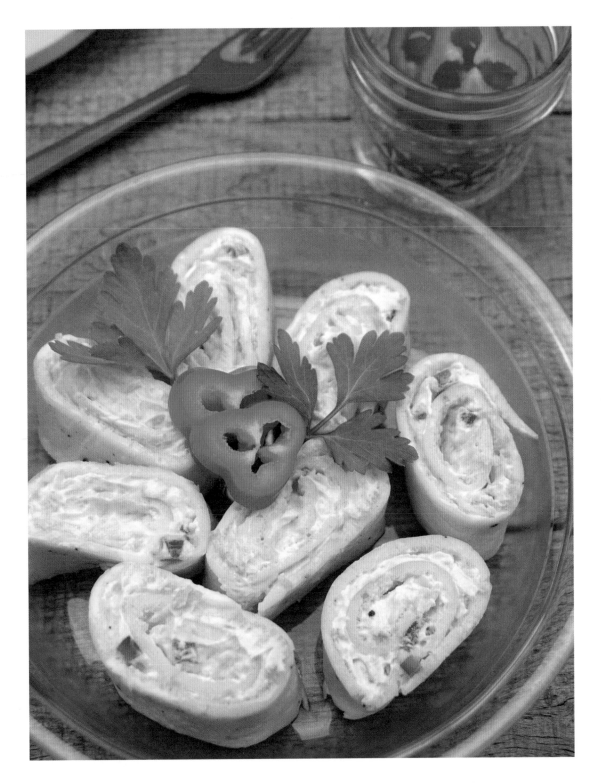

VEGETARIAN

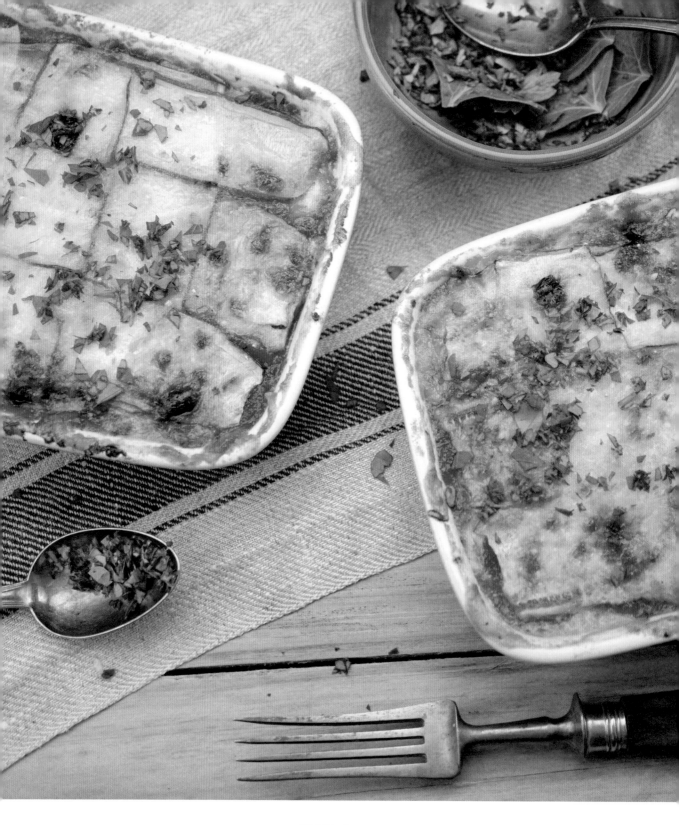

VEGETARIAN

Courgette lasagne

the low-carb way

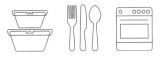

2 eggs
200g (7oz) ricotta
60g (2oz) grated Parmesan,
　plus some extra for scattering
grated zest of 1 organic lemon
salt and freshly ground
　black pepper
250g (9oz) tinned chopped
　tomatoes
1 tsp dried thyme
1 tsp dried basil
1 courgette, sliced lengthways
　into strips with a peeler
200g (7oz) grated Gouda
chopped flat-leaf parsley,
　to garnish (optional)

Preheat the oven to 200°C (400°F/Gas 6). Whisk the eggs in a bowl. Stir in the ricotta, parmesan, and lemon zest. Season the ricotta mixture with salt and pepper.

Stir the chopped tomatoes in a bowl with the thyme and basil, season the tomato sauce to taste with salt and pepper.

Arrange all the ingredients in alternating layers in 2 small ovenproof dishes (about 20 x 10cm/8 x 4in). Start with some courgette strips, then some of the ricotta mixture, scatter with some of the Gouda, and spread some tomato sauce on top. Continue layering the ingredients in this manner, finishing with a courgette layer. Scatter over the Parmesan.

Bake the courgette lasagnes in the centre of the oven until golden brown. Remove from the oven and leave to cool in the dishes then pack into containers. Store in the fridge until ready to eat. If you wish, pack some chopped parsley in a container.

AT WORK — preheat the oven to 200 °C (400°F/Gas 6) and reheat for about 15 minutes. Alternatively, reheat in the microwave until the lasagna is piping hot all the way through. Scatter with chopped parsley, if using.

At home	At work	Serves	Kcal	Protein	Carbs	Fat
30 + 30 mins	15 mins	2	780	58g	13g	48g

Stuffed mushrooms
with spinach and cream cheese

1 tbsp butter
1 shallot, finely diced
400g (14oz) mushrooms
    (preferably not too small),
    stalks removed, plus 2 whole
    mushrooms finely chopped
40g (1¼oz) courgette, cut into
    small cubes
1 garlic clove, crushed
30g (1oz) spinach leaves,
    finely chopped
70g (2¼oz) full-fat cream cheese
salt and freshly ground
    black pepper
10g (¼oz) Parmesan cheese,
    grated

Chop the mushroom stalks and combine them with the 2 chopped whole mushrooms. Melt the butter in a pan and sauté the shallot. Add the chopped mushrooms and the courgette. Add the garlic and the spinach and stir everything together. Add the cream cheese and let it melt. Season to taste with salt and pepper.

Preheat the oven to 220°C (425°F/Gas 7). Line a baking tray with baking parchment. Place the mushroom caps upside down on the baking parchment and fill with the cream cheese mixture. Sprinkle over the Parmesan. Bake the mushrooms in the centre of the oven for 15–20 minutes. Remove from the oven and leave to cool. Transfer to a container and close. Store the stuffed mushrooms in the fridge until ready to serve.

AT WORK — preheat the oven to 220°C (425°F/Gas 7). Reheat the stuffed mushrooms in the oven for about 15 minutes. Alternatively, reheat in the microwave until the mushrooms are piping hot all the way through.

At home	At work	Serves	Kcal	Protein	Carbs	Fat
15 + 20 mins	15 mins	2	265	11g	4g	23g

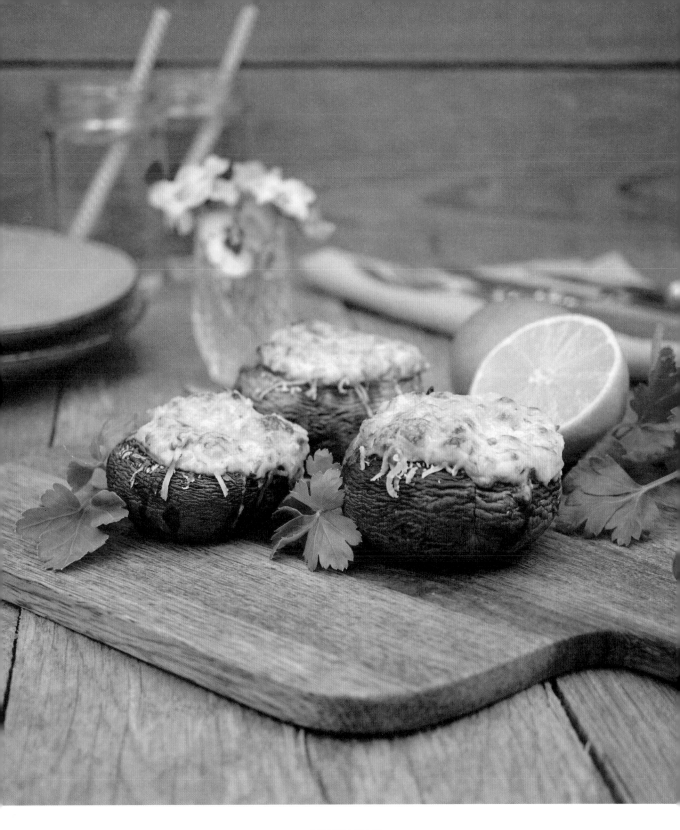

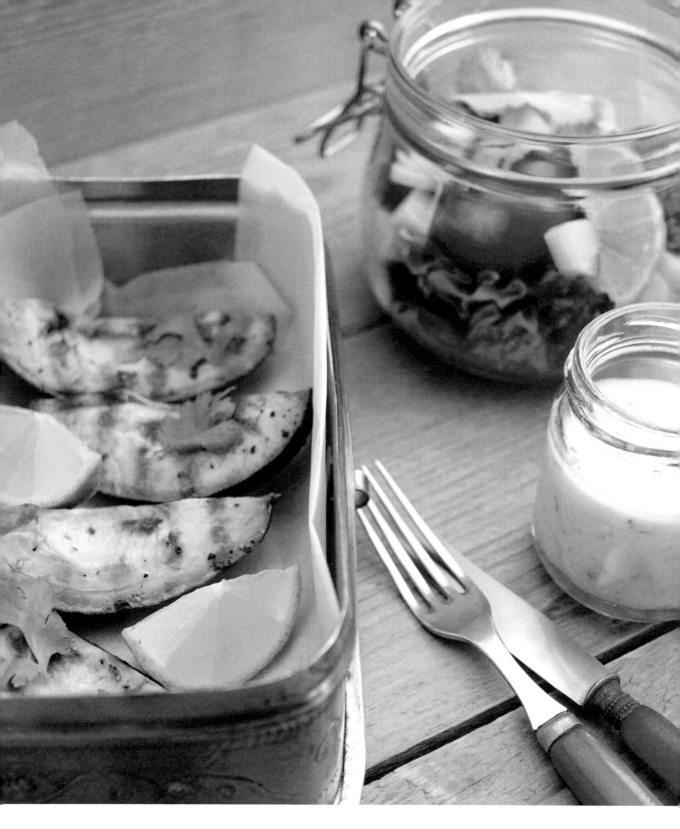

Grilled avocado with salad
and lime dressing

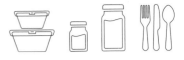

FOR THE SALAD
30g (1oz) mixed leaves
25g (scant 1oz) cucumber,
    peeled and chopped into
    small pieces
3 cherry tomatoes
slices of lime (optional)

FOR THE DRESSING
85g (3oz) yogurt
zest and juice of 1 organic lime
½ spring onion, green section
    only, finely chopped
2 sprigs of coriander leaves,
    finely chopped
salt and freshly ground
    black pepper
agave syrup (optional)

FOR THE AVOCADO
½ tbsp olive oil
1 avocado, pitted, flesh cut
    into 4 wedges
lime wedges (optional)

Place the salad ingredients in a jar, adding some sliced lime if you wish, and close the jar.

To make the dressing, put the yogurt in a bowl and stir in a dash of lime juice. Add the spring onion, coriander, and lime zest and mix together thoroughly. Season the dressing with salt and pepper and some agave syrup, if using. Pour the dressing into a small jar and seal.

For the avocado, put the olive oil on a plate and season with salt and pepper, mixing them together with a fork. Toss the avocado slices in the oil mixture. Heat a griddle pan and fry the avocado slices, fruit-side down, over a high heat, until they have acquired griddle marks. Transfer the avocado to a container, adding some extra lime wedges, if using. Store the dressing and the avocado in the fridge until ready to serve.

At home	At work	Serves	Kcal	Protein	Carbs	Fat
20 mins	0 min	1	310	6g	15g	24g

Pumpkin soup

with aromatic pumpkin seed oil

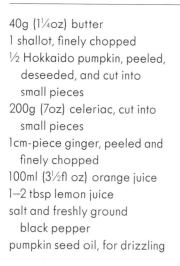

40g (1¼oz) butter
1 shallot, finely chopped
½ Hokkaido pumpkin, peeled,
    deseeded, and cut into
    small pieces
200g (7oz) celeriac, cut into
    small pieces
1cm-piece ginger, peeled and
    finely chopped
100ml (3½fl oz) orange juice
1–2 tbsp lemon juice
salt and freshly ground
    black pepper
pumpkin seed oil, for drizzling

Melt the butter in a large pan and sauté the shallot briefly. Add the pumpkin and celeriac and sauté everything until golden. Deglaze the pan with a dash of water then gradually add 750ml (1¼ pints) water. Add the ginger, cover, and simmer over a moderate heat for 10–15 minutes, until the vegetables are soft.

Remove the pan from the heat and blend the soup using a hand-held blender. Add the orange and lemon juice and stir everything through once more. Season the soup to taste with salt and pepper, transfer to a large jar, and leave to cool. Close the jar and store the soup in the fridge until ready to serve.

AT WORK — reheat the soup, but do not let it boil. Pour into bowls and drizzle with pumpkin seed oil.

OUR TIP — chopped pumpkin seeds also make a great topping for this soup.

At home	At work	Serves	Kcal	Protein	Carbs	Fat
30 mins	10 mins	4	190	3g	18g	12g

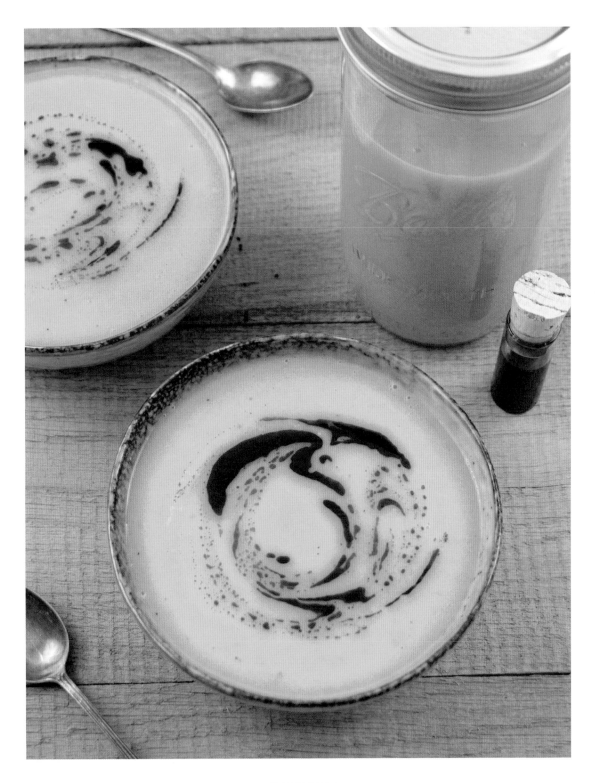

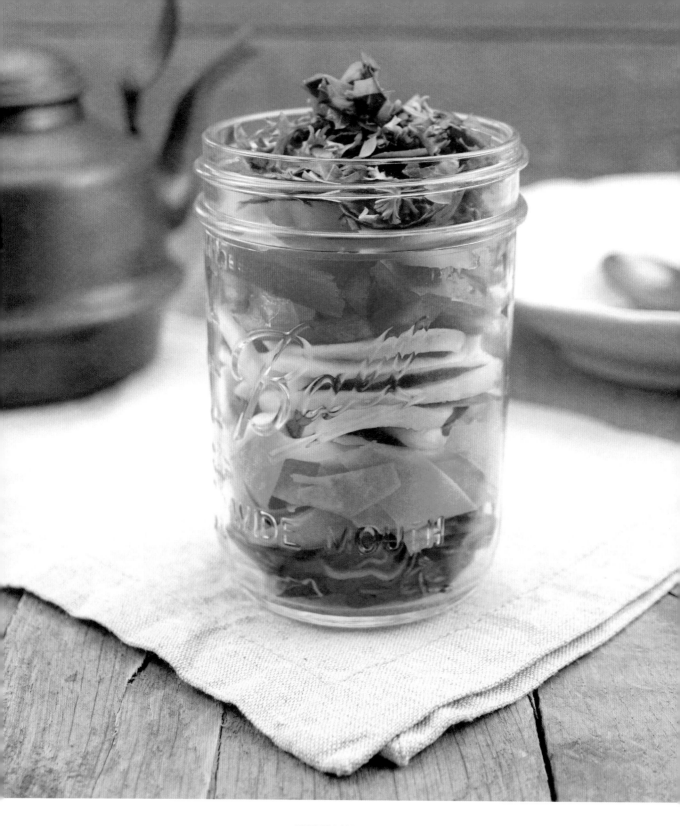

Vegetable noodle soup

with fresh parsley

40g (1¼oz) courgette
1 red cabbage leaf, about
    15g (½oz), thinly sliced
20g (¾oz) squash or pumpkin
    flesh, thinly sliced
40g (1¼oz) red pepper,
    deseeded and thinly sliced
30g (1oz) yellow pepper,
    deseeded and thinly sliced
2 sprigs of flat-leaf parsley
    leaves, roughly chopped
salt and freshly ground black
    pepper (in lidded dispensers)

Using a spiralizer, slice the courgette into long noodles. Wash the red cabbage and slice into thin strips.

Layer up the red cabbage, pumpkin, courgette, and the red and yellow peppers in a jar. Finish with the parsley then close the lid. Store the vegetable mixture in the fridge until ready to serve.

AT WORK — fill the jar with boiling water and leave to steep for around 5 minutes with the lid on. Pour the soup into a deep dish and season with salt and pepper.

At home	At work	Serves	Kcal	Protein	Carbs	Fat
10 mins	6 mins	1	45	2g	8g	2g

Tomato and mozzarella kebabs

with herby fromage frais

FOR THE KEBABS
5 cherry tomatoes, halved
1 mini cucumber, cut into discs
¼ yellow pepper, deseeded and
    cut into 1-cm cubes
sprig of basil leaves
5 mini mozzarella balls

FOR THE FROMAGE FRAIS
4–5 sprigs coriander leaves,
    finely chopped
150g (5½oz) full-fat fromage frais
salt and freshly ground
    black pepper

ALSO
5 small wooden skewers

To make the skewers, slide alternate tomatoes, cucumber, pepper, basil leaves, and mozzarella balls onto the wooden skewers. Put the kebabs into a container and seal.

For the fromage frais, stir the coriander into the fromage frais. Season the herby mix to taste with salt and pepper. Decant into a container, then seal. Store the kebabs and herby fromage frais in the fridge until ready to serve.

At home	At work	Serves	Kcal	Protein	Carbs	Fat
10 mins	0 min	1	282	18g	12g	18g

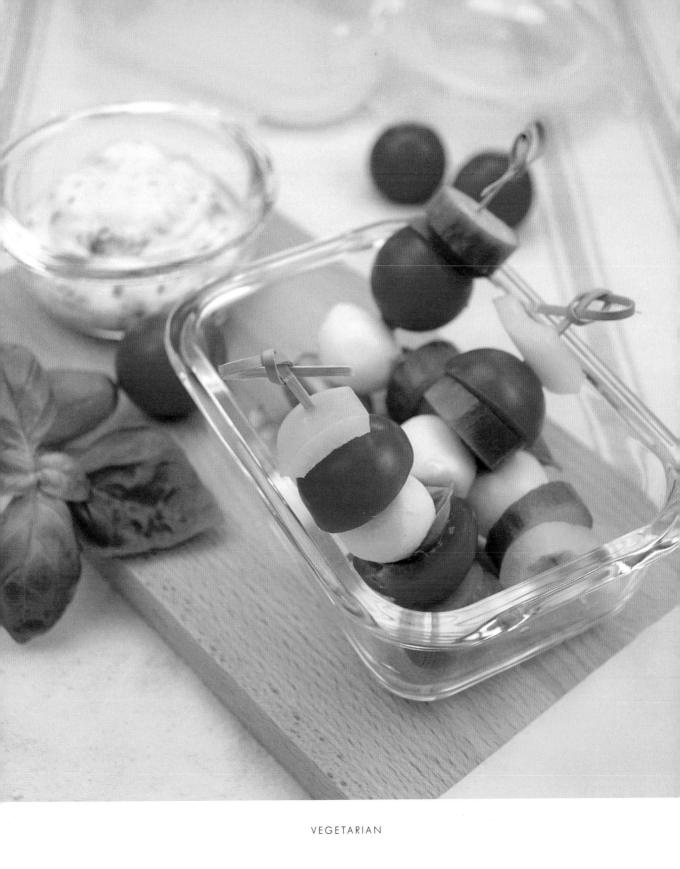

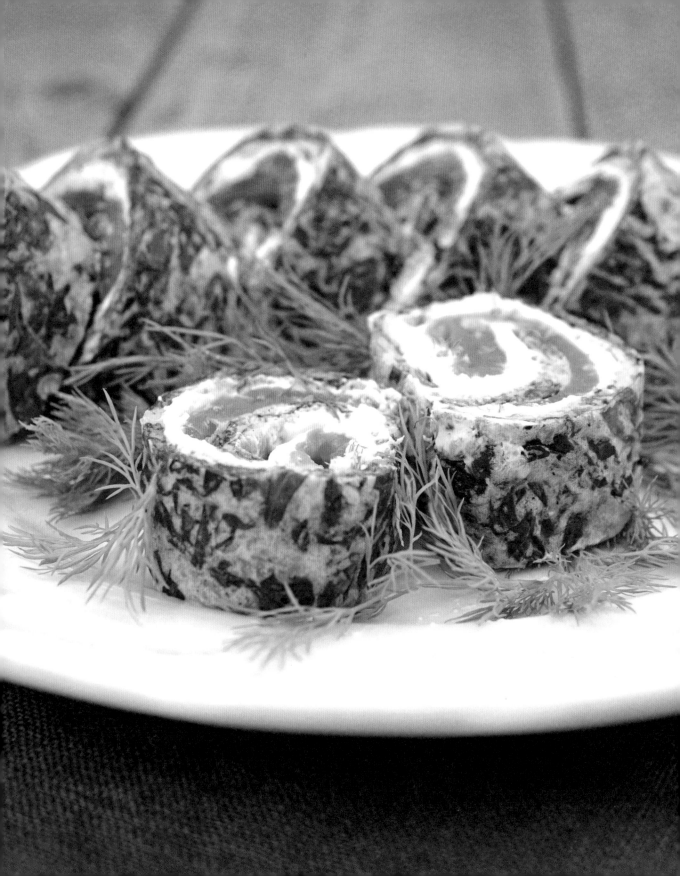

MEAT
AND FISH

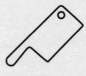

Chicken stock

with spices

1 chicken carcass
3-cm piece ginger, sliced
1 star anise
2–3 cinnamon sticks
salt

Place the chicken carcass in a saucepan with 4 litres (7 pints) water and bring to the boil. Add the ginger, star anise, cinnamon sticks, and salt, cover, and let everything simmer for 1 hour. Then add an additional 1 litre (1¾ pints) water and leave to simmer for a further 2 hours.

Strain the chicken stock through a sieve and decant immediately into sterilized, airtight bottles. Close the bottles immediately and stand them upside down for several minutes, then leave to cool. Alternatively, allow the stock to cool down then freeze it in portions.

At home	At work	Serves	Kcal	Protein	Carbs	Fat
5 + 180 mins	0 min	4	—	—	—	—

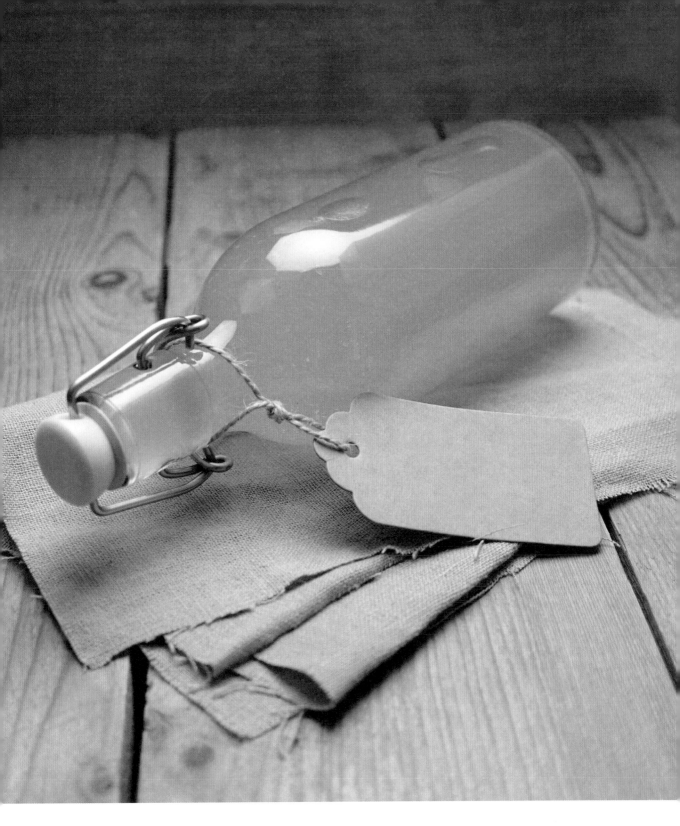

MEAT AND FISH

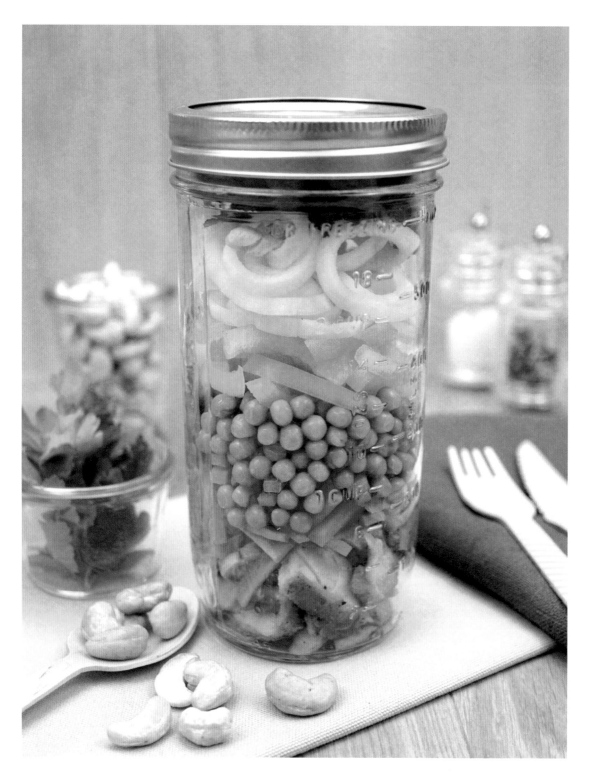

MEAT AND FISH

Life-enhancing soup
with chicken and cashew nuts

1 tbsp coconut oil

1 boneless chicken thigh
(skin on), chopped into
bite-sized pieces

1 broccoli stalk

45g (1½oz) carrot, cut into batons

60g (2oz) peas (freshly podded
or defrosted)

50g (1¾oz) yellow pepper,
deseeded and cut into batons

2 sprigs of flat-leaf parsley
leaves, chopped

1 tbsp cashews, roughly chopped

½ tsp ground cumin

½ star anise

salt and white pepper

Heat the coconut oil in a pan and sauté the chicken pieces for around 5–8 minutes, depending on their size, until cooked. Leave the meat to cool. Use a spiralizer to cut the broccoli stalk into thin noodles.

Layer up the meat, carrot, peas, pepper, and broccoli one after the other in a jar and top with parsley and cashews. Seal the jar. Store the mixture in the fridge until ready to eat. Put the cumin and star anise plus some salt and pepper in a separate container.

AT WORK — add the spice mixture to your jar and pour over boiling water. Close the jar and leave the soup to infuse for 5–7 minutes.

At home	At work	Serves	Kcal	Protein	Carbs	Fat
15 mins	7 mins	1	465	31g	18g	29g

Chicory salad

with chicken

1 tbsp olive oil
50g (1¾oz) chicken breast,
    cut into small pieces
salt and freshly ground
    black pepper
1 orange, divided into segments
1 chicory, thinly sliced
1–2 tbsp pomegranate seeds
handful of mixed leaves,
    roughly chopped
10g (¼oz) beetroot shoots

Heat the olive oil in a pan and sauté the chicken pieces for 5–8 minutes, depending on their size, until cooked. Season with salt and pepper and leave to cool.

Layer up the orange segments, chicory, pomegranate seeds, mixed leaves, chicken, and beetroot shoots one after the other in a jar, then close. Store the salad in the fridge until ready to serve.

OUR TIP — arrange the salad on a plate and drizzle with an aromatic oil, such as grapeseed or pumpkin seed oil.

At home	At work	Serves	Kcal	Protein	Carbs	Fat
15 mins	0 min	1	220	13g	12g	10g

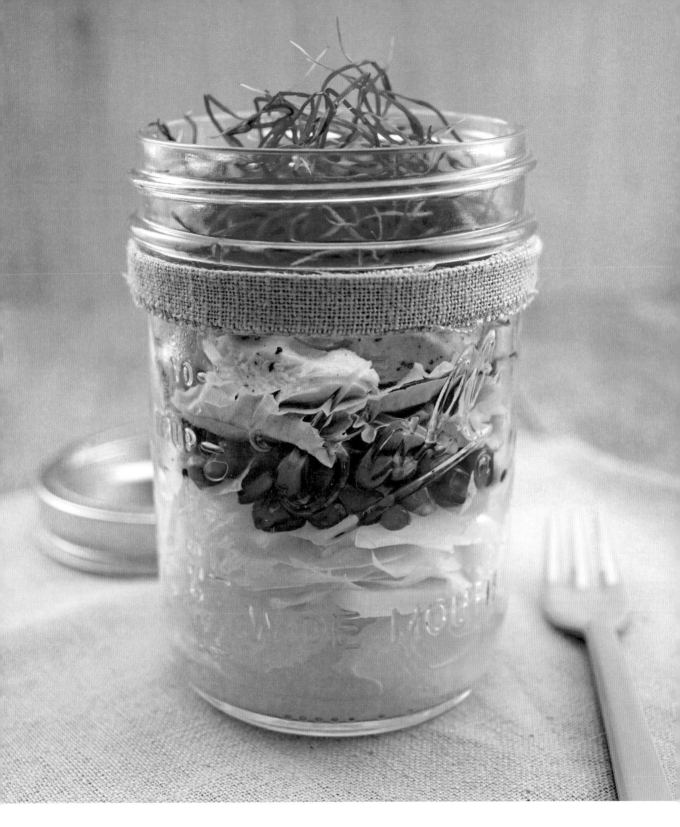

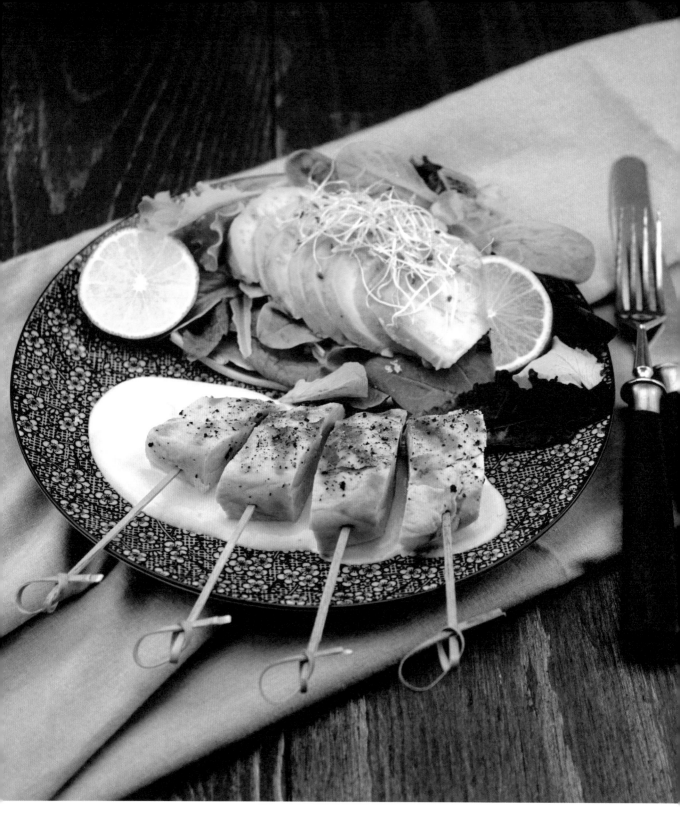

Chicken kebabs

with salad and mustard dressing

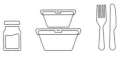

1 chicken breast, about
    150g (5½oz)
salt and freshly ground
    black pepper
½ avocado, pitted and
    flesh sliced
1–2 tsp lime juice
2 handfuls of mixed-leaf lettuce
1–2 tbsp alfalfa sprouts

FOR THE DRESSING
1 tbsp yogurt
½ tbsp full-fat fromage frais
1 tbsp lemon juice
½ tsp medium–hot mustard
salt

ALSO
4 small party skewers

Season the chicken breast with salt and pepper. Heat a griddle pan and fry the chicken for around 5 minutes on each side, until it is cooked through and has acquired griddle marks. While the chicken is cooking, drizzle the avocado with lime juice.

To make the dressing, stir together the yogurt, fromage frais, lemon juice, and mustard. Season the dressing with salt, transfer to a jar, and seal. Store the dressing in the fridge until ready to use.

Remove the chicken from the pan, slice into 4 pieces, leave to cool, then slide onto the party skewers. Put the skewers into a box and close. Put the salad, avocado, and sprouts into a separate box. Store everything in the fridge until ready to serve.

AT WORK — arrange the salad on a plate with the avocado and alfalfa sprouts and season to taste with salt and pepper. Put the dressing on the plate and arrange the chicken kebabs on top.

OUR TIP — if preferred, the chicken can be reheated briefly.

At home	At work	Serves	Kcal	Protein	Carbs	Fat
20 mins	5 mins	1	305	39g	6g	14g

Beef strips

Asian style

juice of ½ lime
1 tsp agave syrup
2 tbsp soy sauce
1 tbsp teriyaki sauce
1–2 tbsp sesame oil
140g (5oz) beef (suitable for
    frying, for example, fillet
    steak), sliced into
    bite-sized strips
1 carrot, cut into discs
1 pak choi, about 200g (7oz),
    quartered
2 mushrooms, thinly sliced
¼ cucumber, peeled, deseeded,
    and thinly sliced
30g (1oz) rice noodles

FOR THE TOPPING
2 sprigs of coriander leaves
1 tbsp chopped cashews
½ tsp white sesame seeds
½ tsp black sesame seeds

Stir together the lime juice, agave syrup, soy sauce, and teriyaki sauce in a little bowl. Heat the oil in a pan and sauté the beef, turning it regularly until brown all over. Add the carrot and pak choi and continue to fry briefly. Then add the mushrooms and cucumber and fry these briefly, too. Stir in the sauce mixture. Put the meat mixture into a container and seal. Leave to cool then transfer to the fridge. Take the noodles with you in a container or in their packaging.

Add the coriander leaves to a jar along with the cashews and sesame seeds.

AT WORK — prepare the rice noodles according to the instructions on the packaging. Heat the meat and vegetables in a pan, then stir in the hot noodles. Serve on a plate and scatter with coriander, nuts, and sesame seeds.

OUR TIP — this recipe can also be prepared completely at home then served cold at work. Instead of rice noodles, you could also use low-carb noodles.

At home	At work	Serves	Kcal	Protein	Carbs	Fat
15 mins	10 mins	2	290	19g	24g	13g

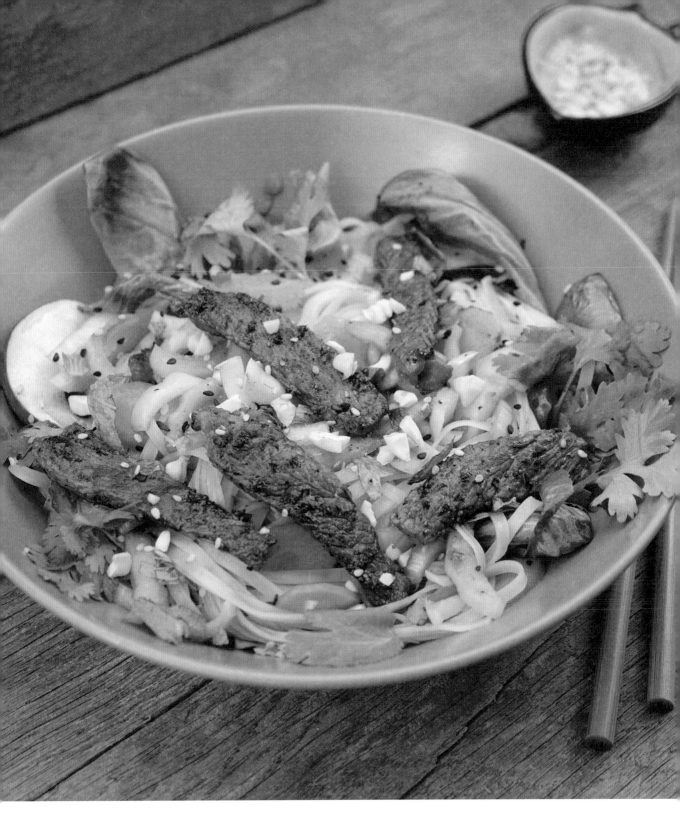

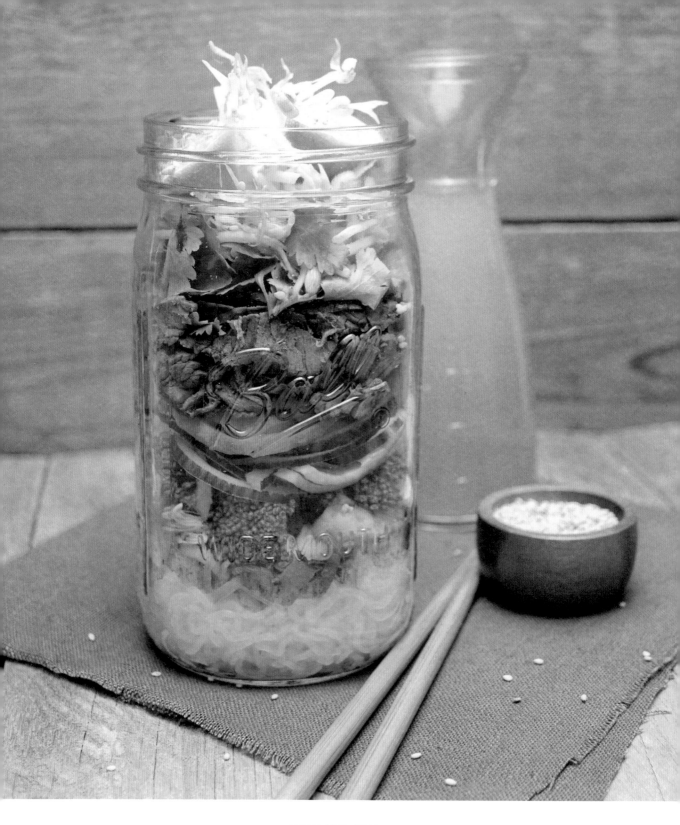

Asian noodle soup

with beef

85g (3oz) shirataki noodles
1 tbsp olive oil
60g (2oz) beef steak
salt and freshly ground
    black pepper
1 spring onion, root discarded
    and white thinly sliced
25g (scant 1oz) small broccoli
    florets
½ red onion, thinly sliced
50g (1¾oz) carrot, peeled
    into long "noodles"
2 sprigs of coriander leaves
1–2 tbsp sprouts or shoots
    (whatever variety you like)
½ organic lime, sliced into
    wedges
500ml (16fl oz) chicken stock
    (see p129)
white sesame seeds for
    scattering (optional)

Rinse off the noodles in a sieve with warm water and leave to drain. Heat the olive oil in a pan and sauté the beef until brown all over. Season the meat with salt and pepper then slice into thin strips.

Layer up the noodles, spring onion, broccoli, red onion, carrots, meat, and coriander in a tall jar, finishing with the sprouts or shoots and lime wedges. Close the jar and store the soup mixture in the fridge until ready to eat. Put the chicken stock and sesame seeds in separate jars. Store the chicken stock in the fridge.

AT WORK — heat the chicken stock and pour over the ingredients in the jar until everything is covered with stock. Close the jar and leave the soup to infuse for 5–8 minutes. Then pour the soup into a bowl and scatter with sesame seeds if desired.

At home	At work	Serves	Kcal	Protein	Carbs	Fat
15 mins	10 mins	1	230	16g	9g	7g

Rainbow rolls
with sweet and sour sauce

FOR THE SAUCE
pinch of agar agar powder
5g ginger, finely chopped
1 garlic clove, crushed
2 tsp sesame oil
3 tbsp cider vinegar
1 tsp lemon juice
1 tsp soy sauce
½ tsp tomato purée
1–2 tbsp agave syrup
½ tsp salt

FOR THE ROLLS
½ avocado, pitted, flesh sliced
1 organic lime
200g (7oz) shirataki noodles
¼ cucumber, cut into thin discs
¼ red pepper, deseeded and
    thinly sliced
¼ yellow pepper, deseeded
    and thinly sliced
30g (1oz) red cabbage leaves,
    finely sliced
1 carrot, thinly sliced
30g (1oz) sugar snap peas
1 tbsp peas (freshly podded
    or defrosted)
salt and white pepper
40g (1¼oz) cooked chicken
2 sprigs of mint leaves
2 sprigs of flat-leaf parsley leaves
9 sheets rice paper (16cm/6½in
    diameter)
1 tbsp white sesame seeds

Stir the agar agar into 2 tablespoons cold water. Put the ginger, garlic, and agar agar water into a saucepan with the sesame oil, vinegar, lemon juice, and soy sauce and bring to the boil. Add the tomato purée and 3–5 tablespoons of water and simmer for about 5 minutes. Season the sauce to taste with agave syrup and salt, transfer to a jar, and seal. Leave to cool. Drizzle the avocado with the juice of half the lime. Chop the cooked chicken into small pieces.

Prepare the noodles according to the instructions on the pack and divide into 9 portions. Season the vegetables with salt and pepper. Mix the noodles with different combinations of vegetables, meat, and herbs. Fill a deep dish with water, soak each of the rice paper sheets for a couple of seconds, as per the instructions on the pack, lay them on a plate, and let each become pliable. Roll up 1 of the noodle mixture portions in each sheet. Scatter the rolls with sesame seeds. Store in a container, with some lime wedges cut from the remaining lime half, in the fridge until ready to serve.

At home	At work	Serves	Kcal	Protein	Carbs	Fat
45 mins	0 min	9 pieces	80	2g	8g	4g

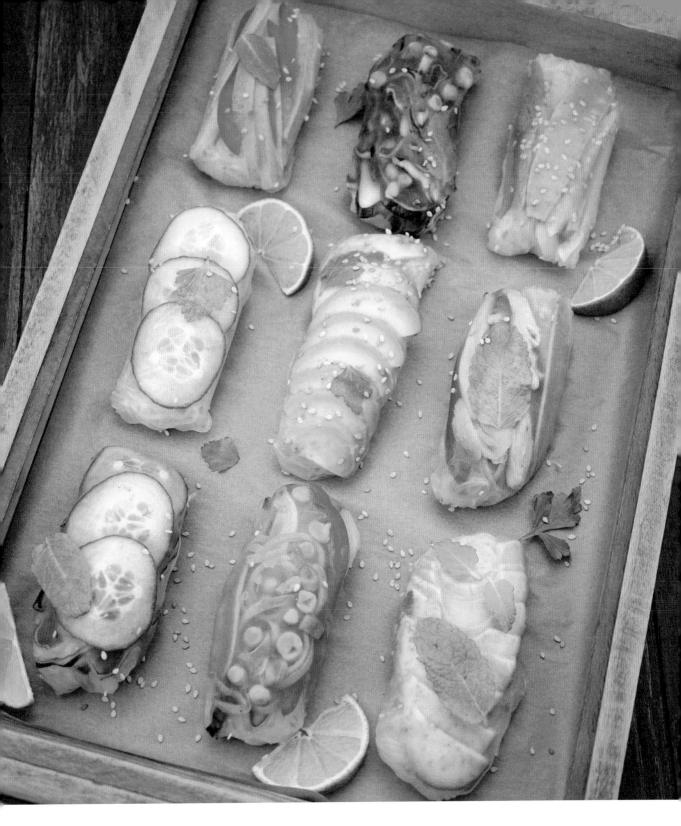

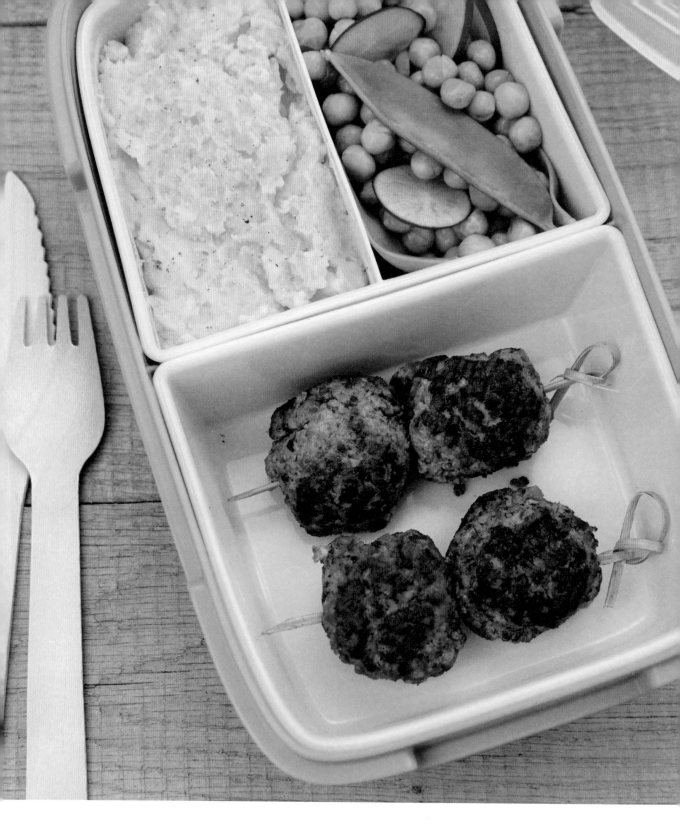

Meatballs with peas

and purée

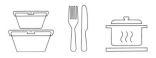

FOR THE MEATBALLS
1 tbsp butter
1 shallot, finely chopped
200g (7oz) minced beef
1 tsp capers, roughly chopped
1–2 sprigs of flat-leaf parsley
    leaves, roughly chopped
1 tbsp yogurt
1 tsp medium–hot mustard
1 egg yolk
salt and freshly ground
    black pepper
1 tbsp olive oil

FOR THE VEGETABLES
4 radishes, sliced
85g (3oz) sugar snap peas
85g (3oz) peas (freshly podded
    or defrosted)
½ tsp cider vinegar
dash of lemon juice

FOR THE PURÉE
1 small parsnip (about 50g/¾oz),
    chopped into small pieces
1 small sweet potato (about
    100g/3½oz), chopped into
    small pieces
freshly grated nutmeg

To make the meatballs, heat the butter in a pan and sauté the shallot until golden. Mix the minced beef in a bowl with the capers, shallots, parsley, yogurt, mustard, and egg yolk. Season the mixture with salt and pepper and shape into little balls. Heat the olive oil in the pan and fry the meatballs for 7–10 minutes, until brown, turning them occasionally. Leave the meatballs to cool and, if desired, slide them onto little party skewers.

Mix all the vegetables together in a bowl with the vinegar, lemon juice, and some salt and pepper.

For the purée, place the parsnip and sweet potato in a pan, just cover with water, put the lid on, and cook for around 10 minutes, until soft. Drain the water. Use a potato masher to turn the vegetables into a purée, season with nutmeg and salt, and leave to cool. Pack up the meatballs, vegetables, and purée into separate containers and seal. Store everything in the fridge until ready to serve.

AT WORK — reheat the meatballs and purée in the pan then arrange on a plate. The vegetable mixture tastes great cold or you can reheat it briefly, if preferred. The cold version is crisper and contains more vital nutrients.

At home	At work	Serves	Kcal	Protein	Carbs	Fat
25 mins	10 mins	2	450	29g	21g	27g

Teriyaki chicken
with cauliflower rice

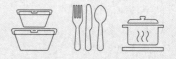

1 tsp coconut oil
1 chicken breast, about
    160g (5¾oz), cut into
    bite-sized pieces
1 garlic clove, crushed
3½ tbsp soy sauce
1 tsp honey
1 tbsp white sesame seeds
½ red onion, sliced into rings
½ red pepper, deseeded and
    finely sliced
½ green pepper, deseeded and
    finely sliced
100g (3½oz) Chinese cabbage,
    cut into 2-cm (¾in) pieces
salt and freshly ground
    black pepper
½ cauliflower, about 400g
    (14oz), finely grated to
    make "rice"
1 tsp black sesame seeds
2 sprigs of coriander

Heat the coconut oil in a pan and sauté the chicken strips on all sides until they are cooked through and have browned slightly. Add the garlic to the pan, along with the soy sauce, honey, and white sesame seeds and sauté briefly. Add the onion, peppers, and Chinese cabbage and continue to fry everything for a further 5–10 minutes, stirring occasionally. Season the teriyaki chicken with salt and pepper, transfer to a container, and leave to cool. Seal the container.

Mix the grated cauliflower rice with the black sesame seeds, transfer to a container, and seal. Pack the coriander in a separate container. Keep all the containers in the fridge.

AT WORK — put the cauliflower rice into a bowl. Heat the teriyaki chicken with the vegetables and arrange on 2 plates. Wash and shake dry the coriander, pluck off the leaves and scatter over the teriyaki chicken.

At home	At work	Serves	Kcal	Protein	Carbs	Fat
15 mins	10 mins	2	295	28g	13g	13g

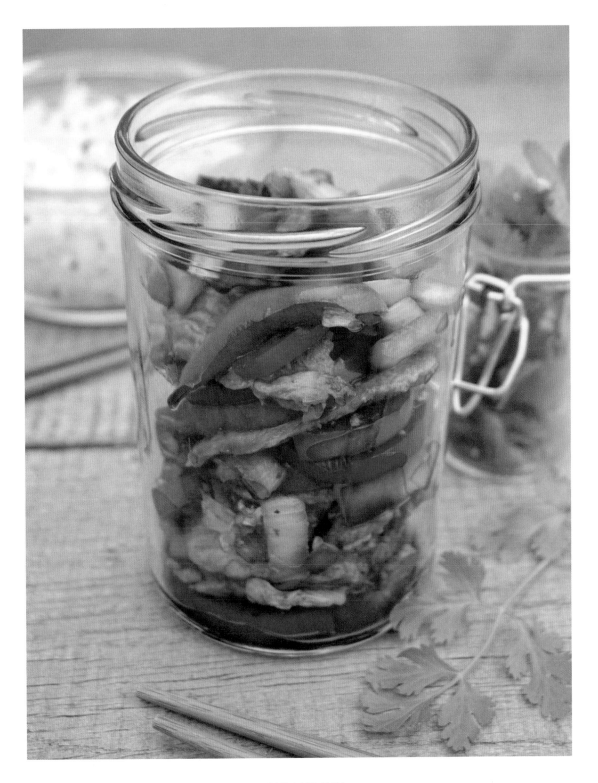

MEAT AND FISH

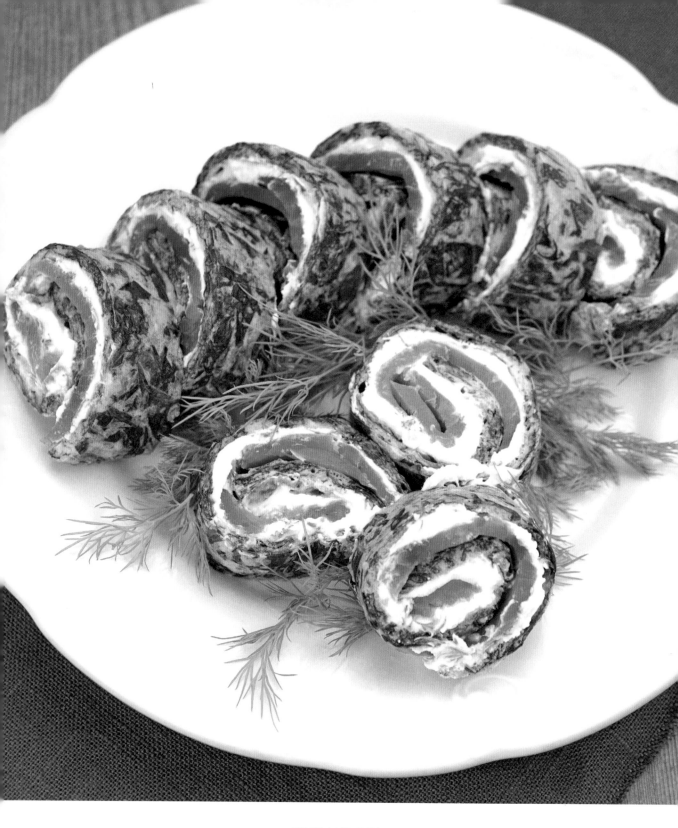

Spinach wraps
with smoked salmon and horseradish

FOR THE WRAPS
250g (9oz) spinach
3 eggs
pinch of grated nutmeg
salt and freshly ground
    black pepper
45g (1½oz) grated Parmesan

FOR THE FILLING
150g (5½oz) full-fat cream
    cheese
zest and juice of 1 organic
    lemon
1-cm (½in) piece ginger,
    finely grated
1 tsp horseradish
salt
3–4 sprigs of dill leaves
150g (5½oz) wild smoked
    salmon

Put the spinach into a steamer over a small amount of water and steam for 3–5 minutes. Remove the steamer section from the pan containing the water, quickly run some cold water through the spinach, and leave to drain.

Preheat the oven to 180°C (350°F/Gas 4). Line a baking tray with baking parchment. Using a hand-held whisk, beat the eggs with the nutmeg and some salt and pepper in a bowl until they are foamy. Stir in the Parmesan and then the spinach. Spread the egg mixture over the baking parchment to create a rectangle and bake in the centre of the oven for 15–20 minutes. Remove from the oven and leave to cool.

While the egg is cooking, stir together the cream cheese, lemon zest, ginger, horseradish, some lemon juice, and salt.

Spread the wrap with the cream cheese mixture, scatter over the dill, and lay the salmon on top. Roll it up carefully and wrap in cling film so that it keeps its shape. Pack into a container and store in the fridge.

AT WORK — slice the wrap using a sharp knife, wiping the knife with a clean, dry cloth after each incision.

At home	At work	Serves	Kcal	Protein	Carbs	Fat
30 mins	1 min	4	295	21g	3g	22g

Griddled prawns

with cucumber and pineapple salad and mango chutney

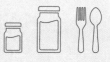

FOR THE CHUTNEY

2 tbsp low-calorie sweetener,
    such as Stevia
1-cm piece ginger, finely
    chopped
½ red chilli, deseeded and
    finely chopped
juice of 1 lime
1 tbsp cider vinegar
½ mango, finely chopped

FOR THE SALAD

2 cucumbers, about 600g
    (2lb 5oz), deseeded and
    finely chopped
1 medium pineapple, about
    600g (2lb 5oz), cored and
    finely chopped
4 sprigs of coriander leaves,
    roughly chopped
4 tbsp lime juice
salt and freshly ground
    black pepper
16 prawns (heads removed,
    shells on)
4 tbsp olive oil

Heat the sweetener in a pan until it becomes liquid. Add the ginger and chilli, deglaze with the lime and vinegar mixture, then simmer everything for a few minutes. Add the mango pieces and leave the chutney to simmer for around 30 minutes, stirring regularly. If it becomes too dry, add some water. Transfer the chutney to a jar and seal. Leave to cool.

For the salad, combine the cucumber, pineapple, coriander, and lime juice in a bowl. Season with salt and decant into jars.

Peel the prawns, make an incision along the backs and remove the intestine. Wash and dab dry the prawns. Heat the oil in a griddle pan, fry the prawns briefly on all sides, and season with salt and pepper. Leave the prawns to cool, then add them to the salad and seal the jars. Store the salads in the fridge until ready to serve.

At home	At work	Serves	Kcal	Protein	Carbs	Fat
60 mins	0 min	4	247	15g	18g	10g

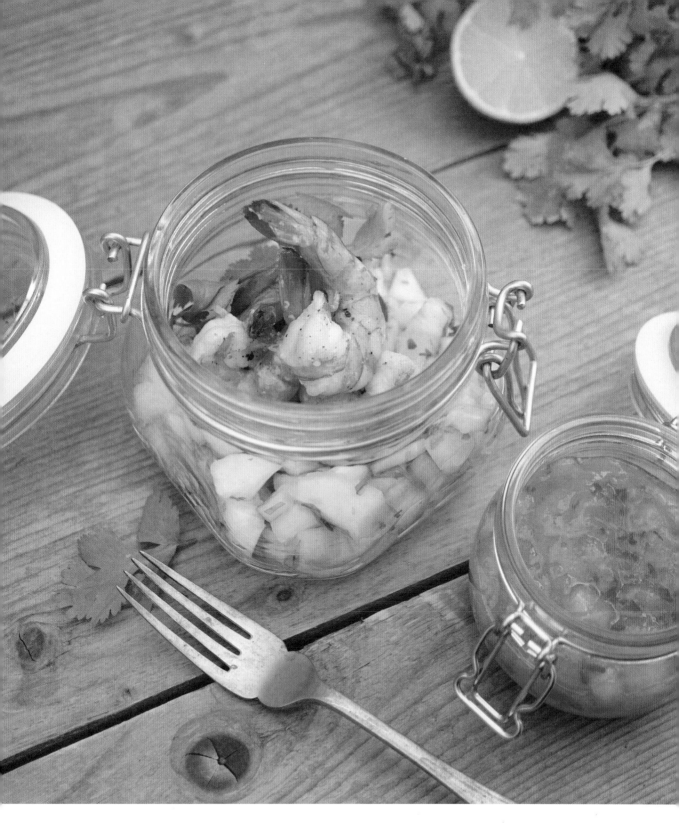

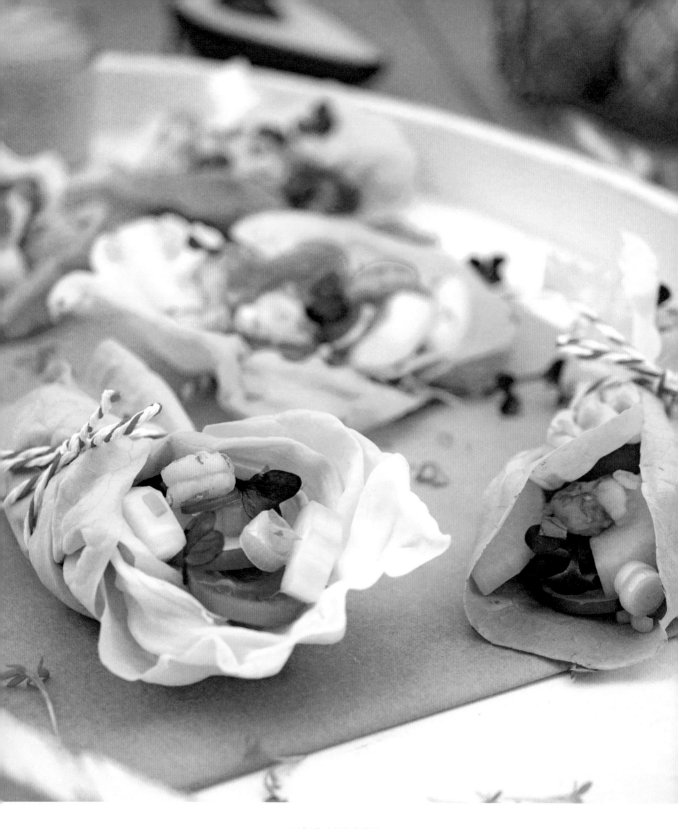

Salad wraps with prawns
and avocado cream

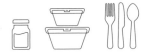

FOR THE SALAD

5 cherry tomatoes

3 radishes

¼ cucumber, peeled and
   chopped into bite-sized pieces

½ spring onion, root discarded,
   white sliced into thin rings

1 chilli, deseeded and finely sliced

125g (4½oz) prawns, cooked
   and peeled

1 tbsp cress (such as garden cress
   or red radish cress), cut

zest and juice of 1 organic lemon

8 large round lettuce leaves

salt and freshly ground
   black pepper

FOR THE CREAM

½ avocado, pitted

juice of ½ lime

2 sprigs of coriander leaves

3 sprigs of dill leaves

3 tbsp yogurt

Put the prepared salad ingredients into a bowl. Add the zest and 1 tablespoon lemon juice and mix everything together. Transfer the mix to a container. Pack the lettuce leaves in a separate container. Seal the containers and store them in the fridge.

To make the cream, add the avocado flesh to a blender beaker along with the lime juice. Add the herbs and yogurt to the avocado and process with a hand-held blender until you have a smooth purée. Season the creamy mix with salt and pepper to taste, transfer to a jar, and seal. Store the cream in the fridge until ready to use.

AT WORK — lay the lettuce leaves out on a plate and distribute the prawn salad between them, seasoning to taste with salt and pepper. Add the avocado cream to the wraps. If desired, tie up the wraps with some thread.

At home	At work	Serves	Kcal	Protein	Carbs	Fat
10 mins	2 mins	3	95	8g	4g	5g

Fishcakes
with pear, fennel, and pea salad

FOR THE SALAD

½ fennel bulb, about
    125g (4½oz), finely sliced
½ small pear, about 60g (2oz),
    peeled, cored, and thinly
    sliced
¼ spring onion, thinly sliced
100g (3½oz) peas (freshly
    podded or defrosted)
2 sprigs of dill leaves, chopped
2 sprigs of coriander leaves,
    chopped
grated zest of ½ organic lemon
1 tbsp lemon juice
2 tbsp orange juice
salt and freshly ground
    black pepper

FOR THE FISHCAKES

225g (8oz) salmon fillet, skin
    removed, cut into small cubes
1 shallot, finely diced
1-cm (½in) piece ginger, grated
½ chilli, deseeded and finely
    chopped
3 sprigs of dill tips, chopped
grated zest of ½ organic lemon
1 tbsp lime juice (or lemon juice)
1 egg yolk
1 tbsp olive oil

To make the salad, combine the fennel, pear, spring onion, peas, herbs, and lemon zest in a salad bowl. Stir in the lemon and orange juice. Season the salad to taste with salt and pepper, transfer to a jar, and seal. Store the salad in the fridge until ready to eat.

To make the fishcakes, combine the salmon, shallot, ginger, chilli, dill, lemon zest, lime juice, and egg yolk in a bowl and season the mixture with salt and pepper. Heat the oil in a pan. Shape 4 equal sized fishcakes from the salmon mixture and fry these in the pan for about 8 minutes, until brown all over, turning them once during cooking. Leave the fishcakes to cool, pack them in a container and store in the fridge until ready to serve.

AT WORK — heat the fishcakes in a pan and arrange them on a plate with the salad.

At home	At work	Serves	Kcal	Protein	Carbs	Fat
20 mins	10 mins	2	395	30g	15g	18g

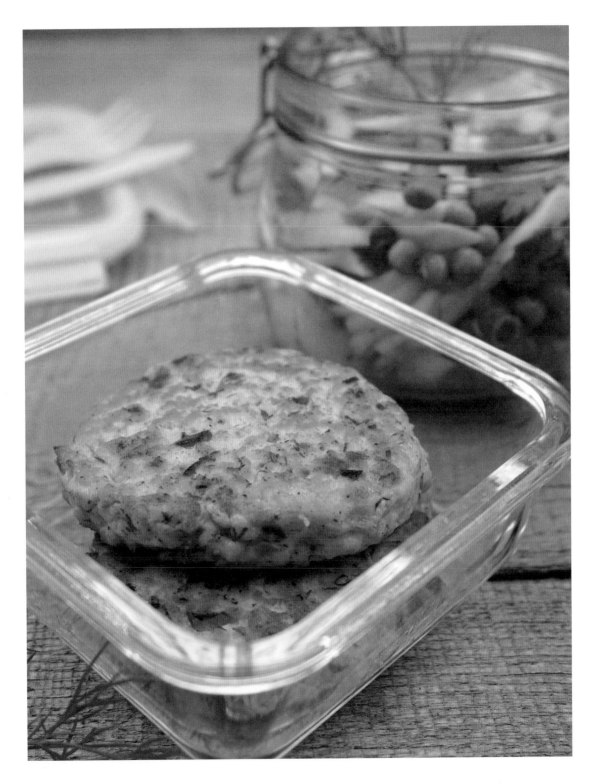

MEAT AND FISH

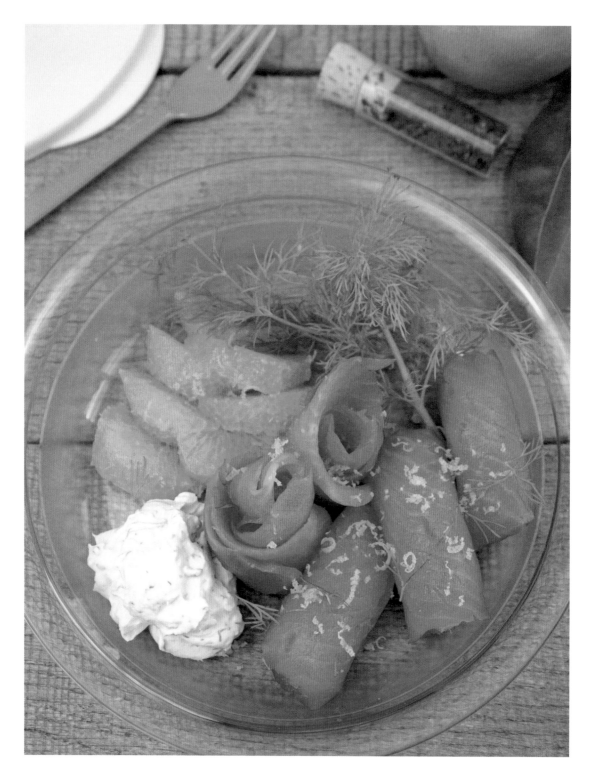

MEAT AND FISH

Fish platter

with gravlax

FOR THE DIP

50g (1¾oz) goat's milk
 cream cheese
2 sprigs of dill tips, finely
 chopped
½ tsp wasabi paste
zest and juice of 1 organic
 lemon
salt and freshly ground black
 pepper (in lidded dispensers)

FOR THE FISH

100g (3½oz) gravlax
2–3 sprigs of dill tips
1 mandarin, pith removed and
 cut into segments
chilli flakes
zest of 1 organic lemon

To make the dip, combine the goat's cheese, dill, and wasabi. Stir the lemon zest and some of the juice into the cheese mixture. Season the dip with salt and pepper, transfer to a jar, and seal. Store the dip in the fridge until ready to use.

For the fish, pack up all the ingredients in containers including the salt and pepper, to take with you. Store the salmon in the fridge until ready to serve.

AT WORK — to prepare the fish, arrange the salmon on a plate with the dill and the mandarin. Sprinkle the salmon with salt, pepper, chilli flakes, and lemon zest and add the dip.

At home	At work	Serves	Kcal	Protein	Carbs	Fat
10 mins	5 mins	1	365	26g	9g	24g

Tuna fish and egg salad

with home-made mayo

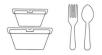

FOR THE SALAD

4 eggs

130g tin tuna in brine
(drained weight)

50g (1¾oz) cornichons, plus
3 tbsp pickling liquid, finely
chopped

½ spring onion, finely sliced

1 celery stalk, finely sliced

60g (2oz) fennel, finely
chopped

2 radishes, finely chopped

30g (1oz) yellow pepper,
deseeded and finely chopped

30g (1oz) red pepper,
deseeded and finely chopped

1 tbsp cider vinegar

100g (3½oz) yogurt

salt and freshly ground
black pepper

FOR THE MAYONNAISE

1 egg yolk

1 tsp medium–hot mustard

1 tsp lemon juice

120ml (4fl oz) oil

FOR THE TOPPING

4 radishes, thinly sliced

2 sprigs of curly leaf parsley,
leaves roughly chopped

4 tsp radish cress

To make the salad, hard boil the eggs in boiling water for 10 minutes, run under cold water, peel, and chop into little pieces. Let the tuna drain in a sieve, then mash it up using a fork.

For the mayonnaise, stir together the egg yolk, mustard, and lemon juice in a bowl with a balloon whisk. Gradually add the oil, one drop at a time at first then in a thin stream, mixing everything thoroughly until you have a creamy mayonnaise. Season with salt and pepper.

Stir together the tuna fish, eggs, vegetables, vinegar, and 3 tablespoons of the cornichon pickling liquid in a bowl. Mix in the yogurt and mayonnaise. Season the salad to taste with salt and pepper, transfer to a container, and seal.

Put the ingredients for the topping into a container. Store the salad and topping in the fridge until ready to serve.

AT WORK — add the topping ingredients to the salad. If you wish, first decant the salad into little bowls.

At home	At work	Serves	Kcal	Protein	Carbs	Fat
20 mins	0 min	4	430	14g	4g	39g

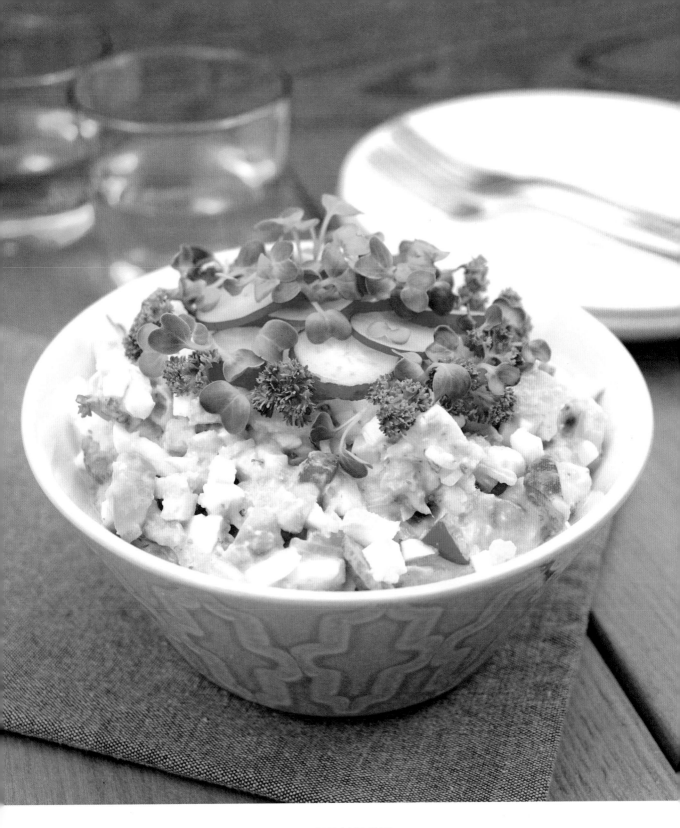

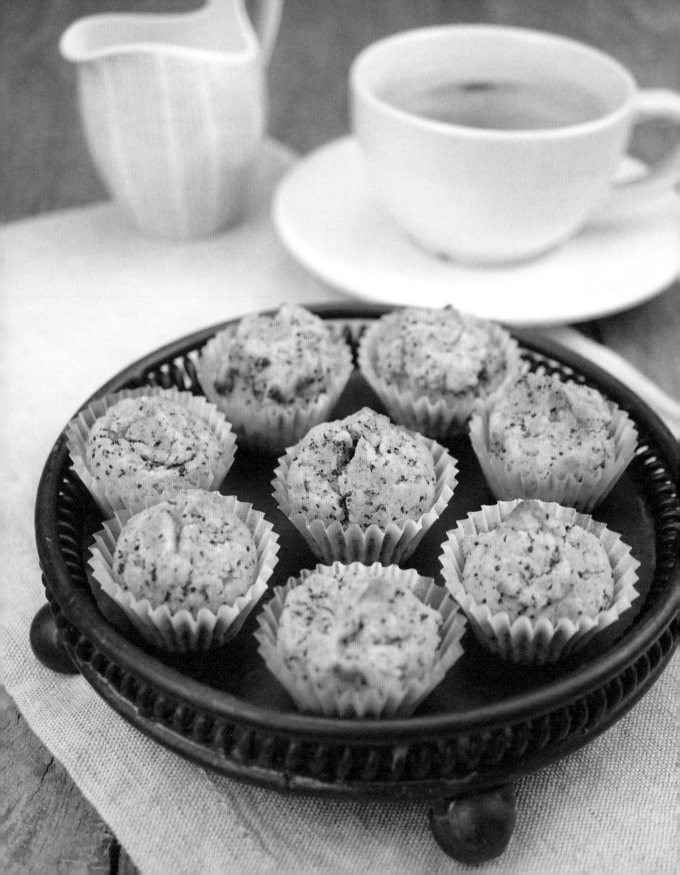

SNACKS

AND CAKES

Low-carb energy bars

with nuts

30g (1oz) walnuts
60g (2oz) almonds
45g (1½oz) pumpkin seeds
3 dates, pitted
1 tbsp cranberries
25g (scant 1 oz) sunflower seeds
seeds from 1 vanilla pod
½ tsp salt
1 heaped tbsp coconut flour

Preheat the oven to 150°C (300°F/Gas 2). Line a baking tray with baking parchment. Roughly chop the walnuts, almonds, and pumpkin seeds in a food processor, then add the dates and cranberries and chop these, too. Combine the nut mixture with the sunflower seeds, vanilla, salt, and coconut flour, kneading everything for several minutes until you have a malleable consistency. Shape the mixture into 6 bars, approximately 1cm (½in) thick, on the tray. Bake in the centre of the oven for 20–30 minutes, until golden brown. Once cooled, store in a tin.

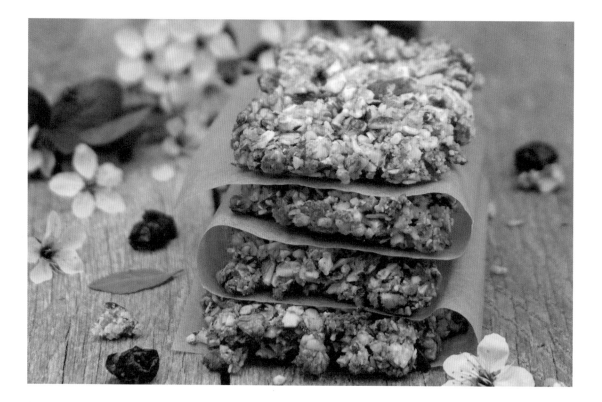

At home	At work	Serves	Kcal	Protein	Carbs	Fat
15 + 30 mins	0 min	6	185	7g	7g	13g

Sesame bars

power snack

15g (½oz) fine oat flakes
75g (2½oz) dates, stoned
10g (¼oz) ground almonds
10g (¼oz) flaked almonds
20g (¾oz) white sesame seeds
30g (1oz) cashew butter
   (see p57)

Lightly toast the oats in a dry pan. Blend the dates in a food processor to create a purée. Use your hands to knead the oats, processed dates, almonds, sesame seeds, and cashew butter to create a dough. Place the dough on a sheet of baking parchment, cover with a second sheet of baking parchment, and roll out to a thickness of approximately 5mm (¼in) using a rolling pin. Cut into 6 bars and let these firm up in the fridge. The bars will keep in a container in the fridge for at least 10 days.

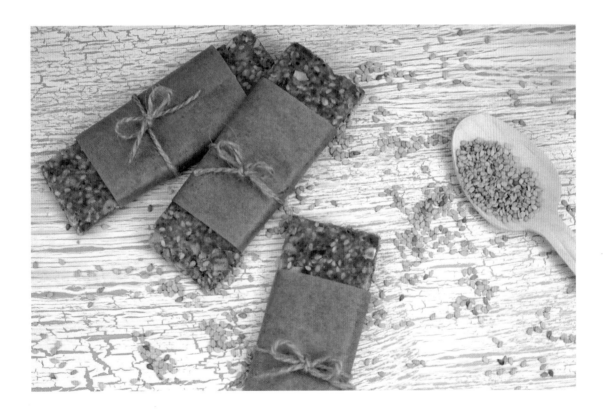

At home	At work	Serves	Kcal	Protein	Carbs	Fat
10 mins	0 min	6	120	3g	12g	6g

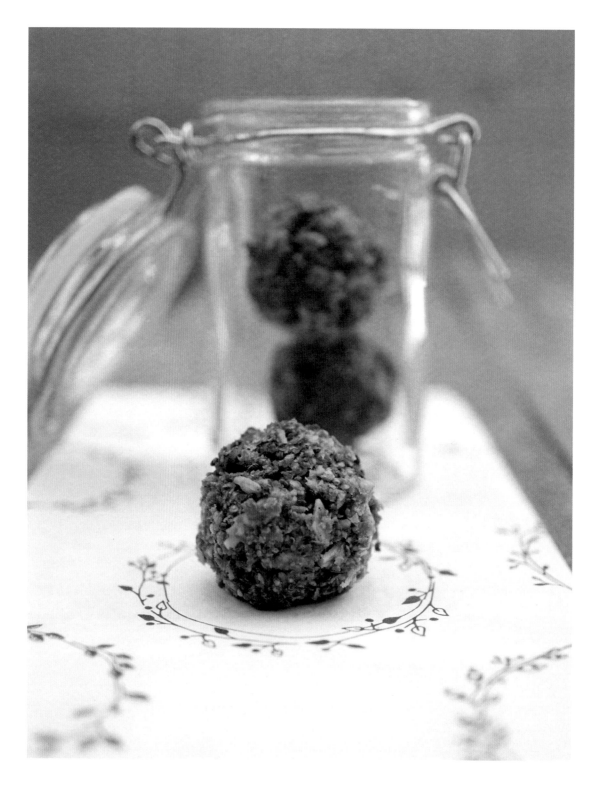

Energy balls
with coconut and vanilla

30g (1oz) spelt bran
20g (¾oz) ground almonds
15g (½oz) flaked almonds
10g (¼oz) chia seeds
½ tsp vanilla powder
1 tbsp cocoa nibs
15g (½oz) coconut sugar
10g (¼oz) coconut flakes
20g (¾oz) smooth coconut oil
2½ tbsp double cream
1 tbsp maple syrup

Preheat the oven to 190°C (375°F/Gas 5). Line a baking tray with baking parchment. Place the spelt bran and ground almonds in a bowl. Crumble the flaked almonds by hand into the spelt mixture and add the chia seeds, vanilla, cocoa nibs, coconut sugar, and coconut flakes. Mix everything together.

In a separate bowl, combine the coconut oil, cream, and maple syrup. Add this mixture to the dry spelt mixture and stir everything well.

Shape the mixture with your hands into walnut-sized balls and place them on the baking parchment. Bake the balls in the centre of the oven for around 10 minutes, until golden brown.

Remove from the oven and allow the balls to cool down on the tray. Store in the fridge in a sealed tin or jar. The balls will keep in the fridge for around 2 weeks.

At home	At work	Serves	Kcal	Protein	Carbs	Fat
15 + 10 mins	0 min	12	75	2g	3g	6g

Fruit slices

in four flavours

BASIC RECIPE
2 tbsp ground nuts
2 tbsp dried fruit
6 round wafer papers
   (5-cm/2in diameter)

BERRY SLICES
2 tbsp ground hazelnuts
1 tbsp fine oat flakes
2 tbsp dried berries
1 date, pitted

APRICOT SLICES
2 tbsp ground almonds
3 dried apricots
1 date, pitted

APPLE CINNAMON SLICES
2 tbsp ground almonds
1 tbsp flaked almonds
1 tbsp coconut chips
4 dried apple rings
½ tsp ground cinnamon

PLUM AND COCOA SLICES
2 tbsp ground almonds
3 prunes
1 tsp raw cocoa powder
1 tsp cocoa nibs
1 date, pitted

Put all the dry ingredients for one recipe into a food processor and chop finely. Add 2 tablespoons of water and mix everything through again. Lay the wafer paper discs out next to each other on the work surface.

Use your hand to shape 3 balls from the fruit mixture. Press each of the balls onto a wafer paper and place a second wafer paper disc on top. Press the balls flat so that they are equal in size and the fruit mixture creates an even layer over the entire disc. The fruit slices will keep for several days in an airtight container.

OUR TIP — the fruit slices will be even tastier if prepared with fruit juice instead of water. If you have a sweet tooth, you could sweeten them to taste with agave syrup or another natural sweetener.

OUR IDEAS FOR OTHER DELICIOUS FLAVOURS — mango and ginger, fig and sesame, date and peanut, or cranberry and coconut.

At home	At work	Serves	Kcal	Protein	Carbs	Fat
10 mins	0 min	3	105	3g	8g	6g

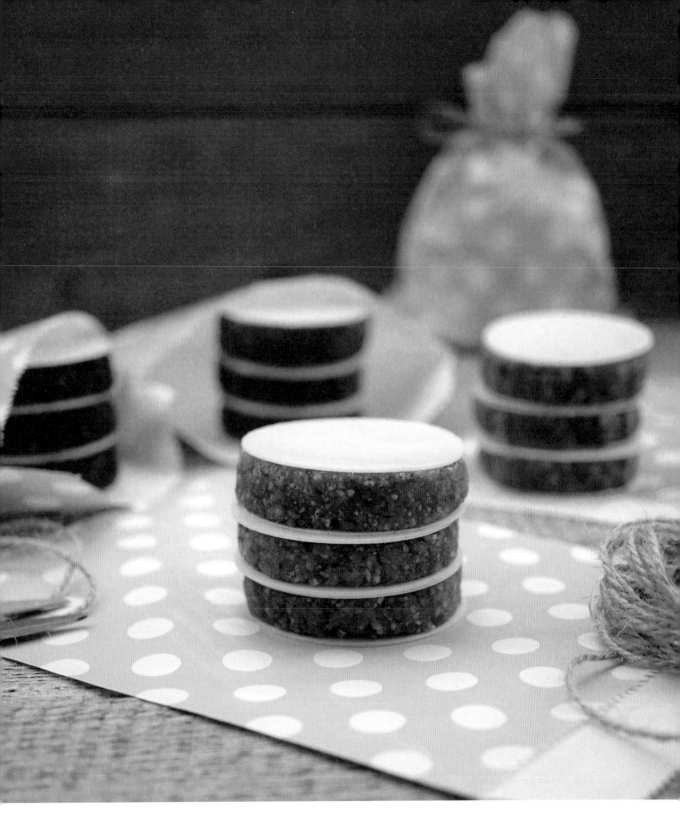

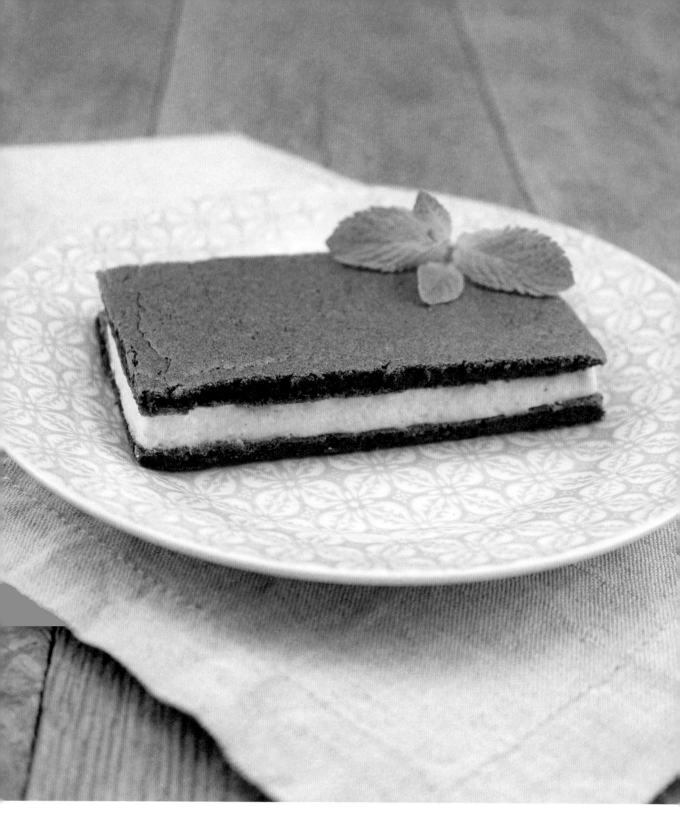

Milk slices

the low-carb way

FOR THE CHOCOLATE DOUGH
1 egg
5g raw cocoa powder
25g (scant 1 oz) full-fat
   cream cheese

FOR THE CREAM
1 very fresh egg white
25g (scant 1 oz) full-fat
   fromage frais
25g (scant 1 oz) mascarpone
1 tbsp coconut protein powder
pinch of vanilla powder

Preheat the oven to 200°C (400°F/Gas 6). Line a baking tray with baking parchment. To make the dough, separate the egg. Use a hand-held whisk to beat the egg white in a bowl until stiff. In a separate bowl, stir together the egg yolk, cocoa, and cream cheese. Carefully fold the beaten egg white into this mixture.

Spread the mixture out evenly on the baking parchment to create a rectangle measuring about 10 x 20cm (4 x 8in), and bake in the centre of the oven for around 10 minutes. Remove from the oven and leave to cool.

To make the cream filling, beat the egg white until stiff. Combine the fromage frais and mascarpone in a bowl. Stir in the protein powder and vanilla. Fold the beaten egg white into the cream and leave the mixture to stand briefly.

Cut 2 equal-sized rectangles from the chocolate slab. Put the cream on one rectangle and spread it out evenly. Place the second rectangle on top of the cream and press down slightly. Put the milk slice into a tin and seal. Store in the fridge until ready to eat.

OUR TIP — if the low-carb milk slice is being prepared in the evening and won't be eaten until the following day, we recommend waiting to spread on the cream until just before you are ready to eat.

At home	At work	Serves	Kcal	Protein	Carbs	Fat
20 + 10 mins	0 min	1	379	33g	5g	25g

Apple and orange muffins
with quinoa

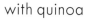

50g (1¾oz) quinoa
100g (3½oz) coconut oil
50g (1¾oz) low-calorie
   sweetener, such as Stevia
1 egg
100g (3½oz) spelt flour with
   a high gluten content
75g (2½oz) wholemeal
   spelt flour
25g (scant 1oz) coconut flour
1 tsp baking powder
150–200ml (5–7fl oz) almond
   milk (see p22, or shop-bought)
2 small apples, peeled,
   cored, and chopped into
   small pieces
1 orange, pith removed and
   chopped into small pieces

ALSO
1 x 12 hole muffin tray
12 paper muffin cases

Preheat the oven to 200°C (400°F/Gas 6). Wash the quinoa in a sieve under running water. Transfer it to a small pan, cover with water, and simmer uncovered for 8–10 minutes, until soft. Insert a paper case into each of the muffin tin holes.

Melt the coconut oil in a pan over a low heat. Place the sweetener, egg, and quinoa in a bowl and stir in the melted coconut oil. In a separate bowl, combine both types of spelt flour, the coconut flour, and baking powder. Add the flour mixture to the coconut oil and egg mixture. Using a hand-held whisk, gradually beat in sufficient almond milk to create a thick batter. Finally, fold in the apple and orange pieces with a spoon. Distribute the batter evenly between the paper cases.

Bake the muffins in the centre of the oven for 20 minutes. Then insert a skewer to see if they are done: as long as no batter sticks to the inserted wooden skewer the muffins are ready. Otherwise, cook for around another 5 minutes. Remove from the oven and leave the muffins to cool for about 5 minutes in the tin. Then lift them out and allow to cool on a wire rack. Pack them up in a container to take with you.

At home	At work	Serves	Kcal	Protein	Carbs	Fat
20 + 25 mins	0 min	12	167	4g	13g	10g

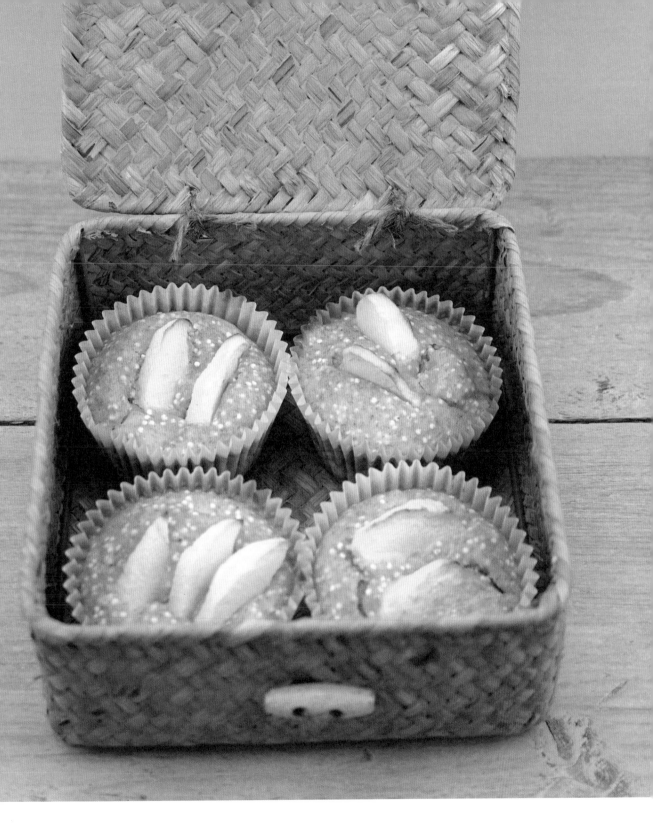

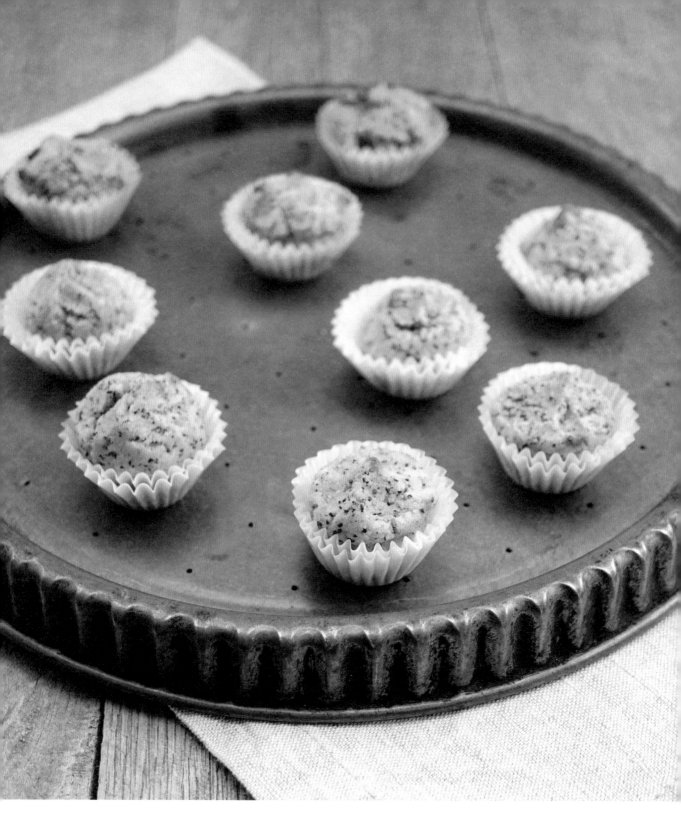

Mini muffins

with poppy seeds and lemon

45g (1½oz) butter
grated zest of 2 organic lemons
2 eggs
30g (1oz) coconut flour
15g (½oz) low-calorie
    sweetener such as Stevia
1 tbsp poppy seeds
pinch of bicarbonate of soda
pinch of vanilla powder
pinch of ground turmeric
pinch of salt

ALSO
32 mini muffin paper cases

Preheat the oven to 190°C (375°F/Gas 5). Put one paper case inside another and place on a baking tray. Melt the butter in a small pan over a low heat then stir in the lemon zest.

Place the eggs, coconut flour, sweetener, poppy seeds, bicarbonate of soda, vanilla, turmeric, and salt in a bowl and stir in the butter mixture with a wooden spoon.

Distribute the mixture between the paper cases, using around 1 tbsp for each muffin. Bake the muffins in the centre of the oven for 5 minutes. Then lower the oven temperature to 160–170°C (275–300°F/Gas 1–2) and cook the muffins for an additional 5–8 minutes, until done.

Remove the muffins from the baking tray and leave to cool on a wire rack. Pack them up in a container to take with you.

OUR TIP — the lemon flavour in the muffins will be particularly enhanced if the zest is completely fresh and added immediately to the warm butter.

At home	At work	Serves	Kcal	Protein	Carbs	Fat
10 + 13 mins	0 min	16	45	2g	1g	4g

Blueberry vanilla cake

for coffee mornings

50g (1¾oz) butter
2–3 tbsp blueberries
(fresh or frozen)
2 eggs
20g (¾oz) xylitol sweetener
30g (1oz) erythritol sweetner
85g (3oz) almond flour
½ tsp cream of tartar
1 tsp vanilla powder
60g (2oz) coconut fat (the
firm layer from a tin of
coconut milk)
sweetener substitute for icing
sugar (optional)
edible blossom (optional)

ALSO

1 springform tin (16–18cm/
6½–7in diameter)
fat for the tin

Preheat the oven to 200°C (400°F/Gas 6). Grease the springform tin. Melt the butter in a small pan over a low heat. Wash the fresh blueberries and leave to drain.

Beat the eggs in a bowl using a hand-held whisk until they are foamy. Add the sweeteners and whisk everything until pale and creamy.

Combine the almond flour, cream of tartar, and vanilla in a large bowl. Add the butter and coconut fat and stir. Fold in the egg and sweetener mixture. Finally, add the blueberries to the mix (there is no need to defrost frozen berries) and stir everything through once more.

Transfer the mixture to the springform tin and bake in the centre of the oven for 30 minutes. Test with a skewer to see if it is done: as long as none of the mixture sticks to the inserted wooden skewer, the cake is ready. Otherwise, continue to cook for a further 10–15 minutes.

Remove from the oven and allow the cake to rest in the tin for around 10 minutes. Release the cake from the tin and leave to cool on a wire rack. Dust with the icing sugar substitute, if using, and decorate with edible flowers, if using.

At home	At work	Serves	Kcal	Protein	Carbs	Fat
15 + 45 mins	0 min	8	130	6g	3g	9g

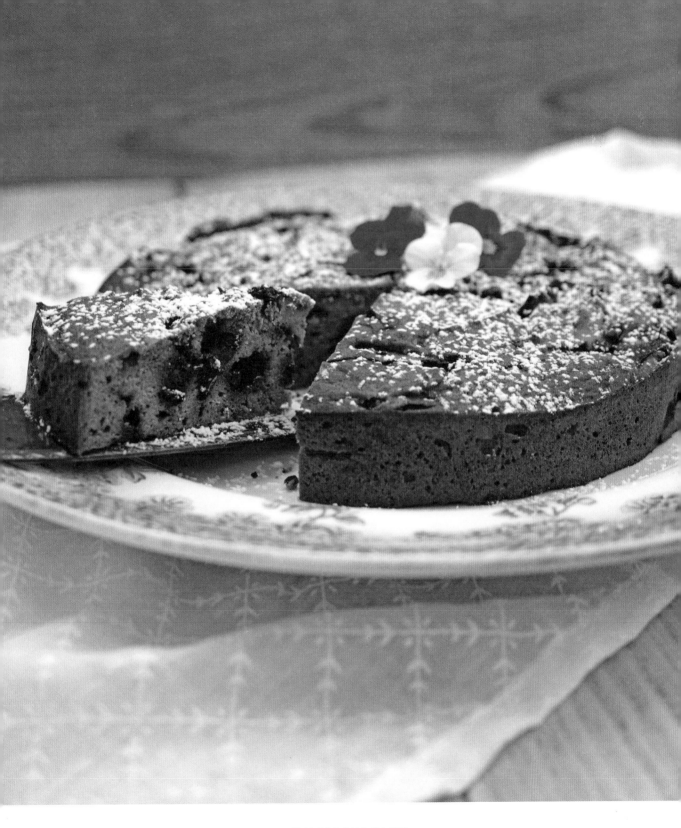

Strawberry rounds

with meringue

2 egg whites
25g (scant 1oz) low-calorie
    sweetener such as Stevia
pinch of salt
30g (1oz) ground almonds
½ tsp vanilla powder
1 tsp locust bean gum
8 strawberries

Preheat the oven to 160°C (325°F/Gas 3). Line a baking tray with baking parchment. Place 1 egg white in a bowl over hot water with 15g (½oz) sweetener and the salt, and beat until stiff. Fold in the almonds, vanilla, and locust bean gum. Shape 4 balls and press flat on the baking tray. Bake in the centre of the oven for 15–20 minutes. Beat the other egg white with 10g (¼oz) sweetener over the bain-marie until stiff. Halve the strawberries and put these and the meringue on top of each cooked disc and cook for 15 minutes.

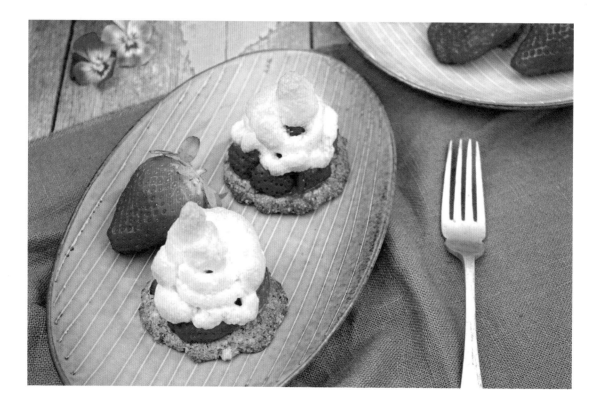

At home	At work	Serves	Kcal	Protein	Carbs	Fat
20 + 35 mins	0 min	4	80	4g	2g	4g

Low-carb cookies
with almonds

1 egg
50g (1¾oz) almond butter
30g (1oz) low-calorie
   sweetener such as Stevia
75g (2½oz) ground almonds

Preheat the oven to 190°C (375°F/Gas 5). Line a baking tray with baking parchment. Beat the egg in a bowl until foamy, then stir in the almond butter and sweetener. Add the ground almonds and combine everything. Use a teaspoon to make approximately 15 little blobs of mixture on the baking parchment. Bake the cookies in the centre of the oven for 10–15 minutes, until a pale golden colour. Remove from the tray and leave to cool on a wire rack. Store in a container.

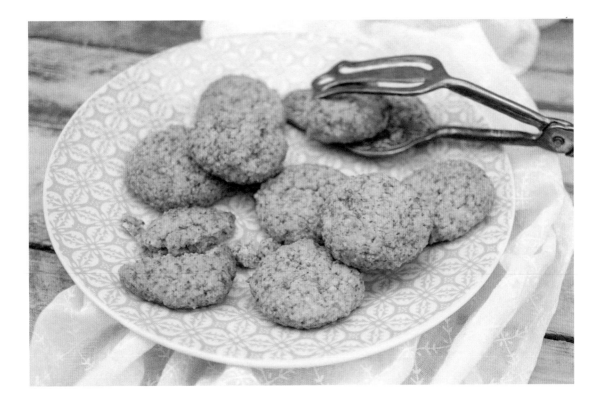

At home	At work	Serves	Kcal	Protein	Carbs	Fat
10 + 15 mins	0 min	15	65	2g	1g	4g

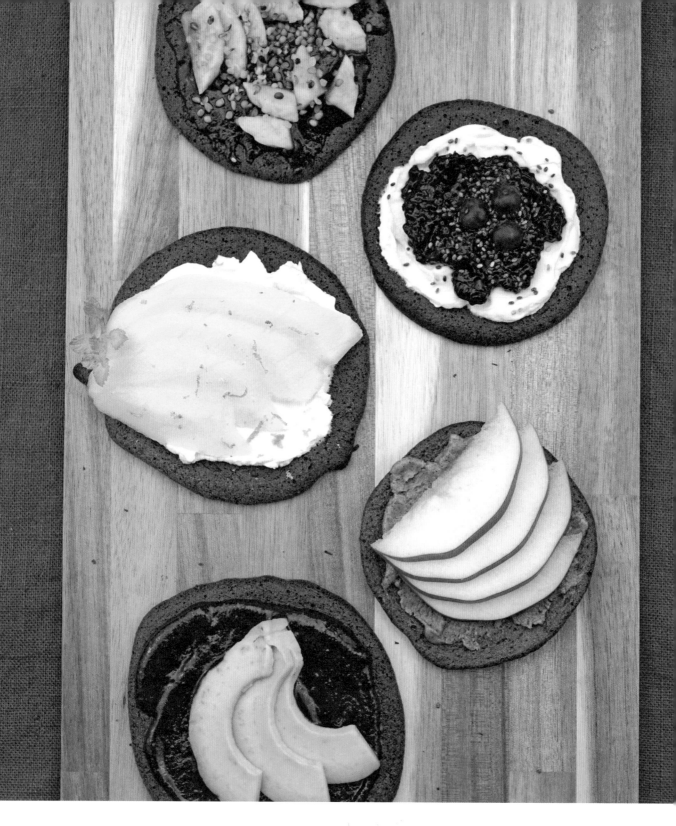

Chocolate "oopsies"
with toppings

FOR THE OOPSIES
2 eggs
salt
40g (1¼oz) full-fat cream cheese
15g (½oz) raw cocoa powder
dash of agave syrup
cream cheese, fromage frais,
    or spread
seeds and fruits, cut into
    bite-sized pieces (optional)

Preheat the oven to 190°C (375°F/Gas 5). Line 2 baking trays with baking parchment. Separate the eggs. In a bowl, beat the egg whites with a pinch of salt until stiff. Combine the egg yolks with the cream cheese, cocoa, agave syrup, and an extra pinch of salt. Fold in the beaten egg whites. From this mixture, create 10 discs on the trays – not too close together, otherwise the oopsies will merge. Bake in the centre of the oven for 10–15 minutes. Leave to cool and pack up in a container. Put the cream cheese, fromage frais, or spread and seeds and fruits, if using, into containers.

At home	At work	Serves	Kcal	Protein	Carbs	Fat
15 + 5 mins	0 min	10	30	2g	1g	2g

CINNAMON SPREAD
50g (1¾oz) almond butter
½ tsp ground cinnamon
½ tsp vanilla powder
1 tsp agave syrup
grated nutmeg

Place all the ingredients in a blender beaker and use a hand-held blender to process everything to a smooth purée. Transfer the cinnamon spread to a jar and seal. Store the cinnamon spread in the fridge, where it will keep for up to 10 days.

At home	At work	Serves	Kcal	Protein	Carbs	Fat
5 mins	0 min	5	70	2g	2g	6g

CHOCO HEMP CREAM
60g (2oz) coconut oil
20g (¾oz) cocoa powder
30g (1oz) hulled hemp seeds
agave syrup, to taste

Melt the coconut oil in a pan over a low heat. Put the oil into a blender beaker with the cocoa and hemp seeds and use a hand-held blender to process to a creamy consistency. Sweeten the cream to taste with agave syrup, transfer to a jar, and leave to cool. Close the jar and store in a cold place. The cream will keep in the fridge for at least 1 week.

At home	At work	Serves	Kcal	Protein	Carbs	Fat
10 mins	0 min	10	80	2g	1g	7g

Coconut waffles

with icing sugar substitute and berries

30g (1oz) butter
1 tbsp coconut oil
2 eggs
60g (2oz) full-fat fromage frais
3 heaped tbsp coconut
   protein powder
1 level tsp cream of tartar
some icing sugar substitute
fruits (optional)

ALSO
waffle iron

Melt the butter and coconut oil in a pan over a low heat. Whisk the eggs in a bowl. Add the fromage frais, butter, and coconut oil and stir everything well. Mix in the protein powder and cream of tartar. If the mixture is too thick, stir in an additional 1–2 tablespoons water to create a smooth, thick batter.

Preheat the waffle iron. For each waffle, put a ladle of batter onto the waffle iron and cook until golden brown. Leave the waffles to cool on a wire rack and pack into containers.

AT WORK — dust the waffles with the icing sugar substitute and top with fruit, if using.

OUR TIP — if you like, you can create several portions of the batter at home then take this into work along with your waffle iron. Freshly cooked waffles are always the best!

At home	At work	Serves	Kcal	Protein	Carbs	Fat
15 mins	1 min	2	391	35g	4g	25g

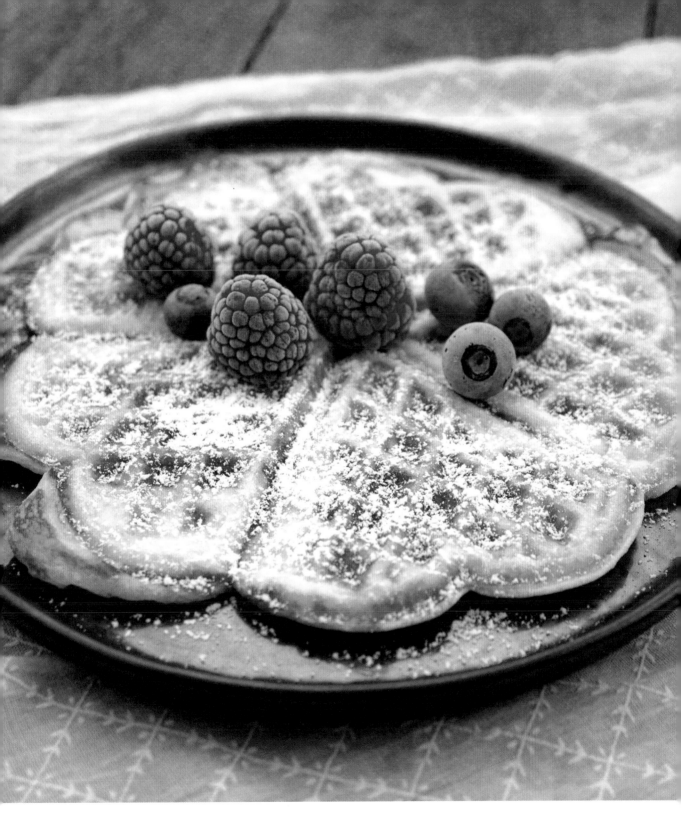

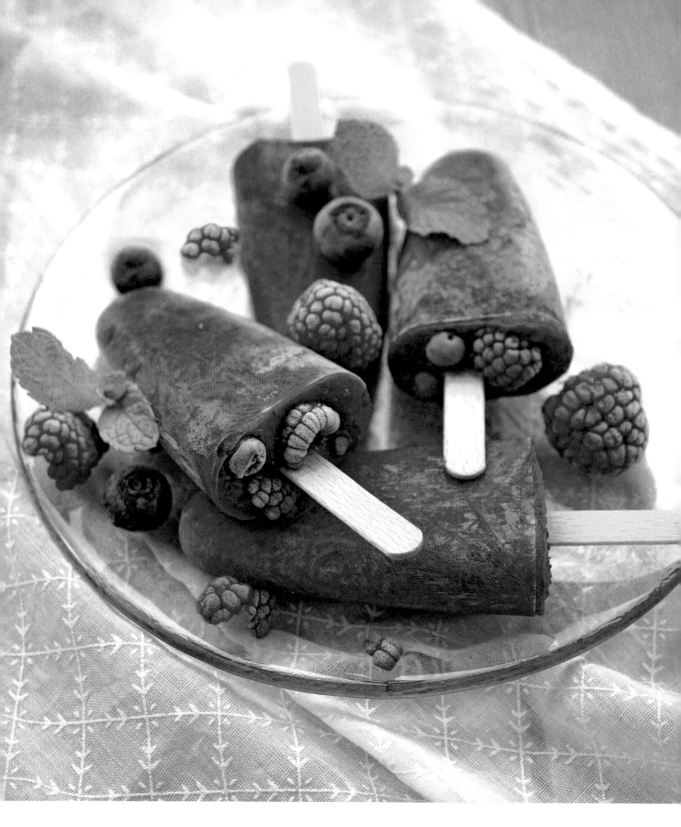

Frozen berries
ice lollies

100g (3½oz) mixed berries
   (fresh or frozen)
1 tbsp yogurt
150ml (5fl oz) milk
low-calorie sweetener, such
   as Stevia, to taste
1 tbsp chia seeds

ALSO
6 ice lolly moulds
6 lolly sticks

Put the yogurt, milk, and about 75g (2½oz) of berries (frozen berries do not have to be thawed) into a food processor and blend until smooth. Add the remaining berries to the purée and sweeten to taste with the sweetener.

Pour the purée into an airtight and leakproof container and close. Store in the fridge until you are ready to use.

AT WORK — stir the chia seeds into the berry mixture. Pour the cold mix into the lollipop moulds and insert 1 lolly stick into each. They will need at least 2 hours in the freezer before they are ready.

At home	At work	Serves	Kcal	Protein	Carbs	Fat
5 mins	5 + 120 mins	6	30	2g	2g	1g

Pecan candies

with coconut

45g (1½oz) pecans (plus
  6 pecans to decorate)
1 tbsp coconut oil
40g (1¼oz) dates, pitted
½ tsp vanilla powder

Finely grind the pecans in a food processor. Melt the coconut oil in a small pan over a low heat. Add the dates, vanilla, and melted coconut oil to the ground nuts and process everything together until you have a fine consistency.

Use your hands to shape the nut mixture into a ball and place this on a sheet of baking parchment. Lay a second sheet of baking parchment on top and use a rolling pin to roll the mixture out to an approximately 1-cm (½in) thick rectangle. Use a knife or cookie cutter to cut or stamp out squares measuring roughly 3 x 3cm (1½ x 1½in).

Place 1 pecan nut on each square and press in slightly. Let the candies firm up in the fridge. Store in a container until ready to eat. The pecan candies will keep for at least 1 week in the fridge.

At home	At work	Serves	Kcal	Protein	Carbs	Fat
10 mins	0 min	6	100	1g	5g	8g

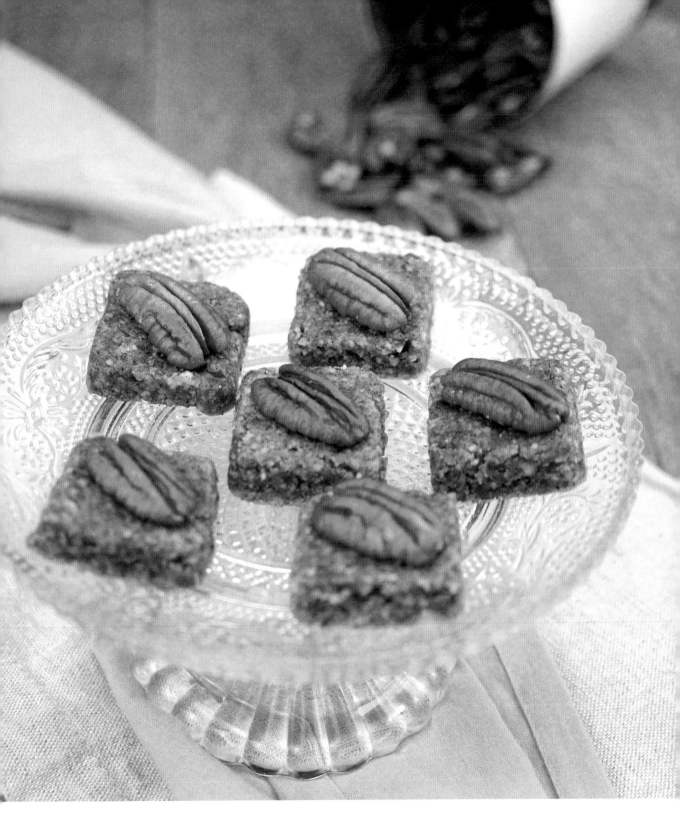

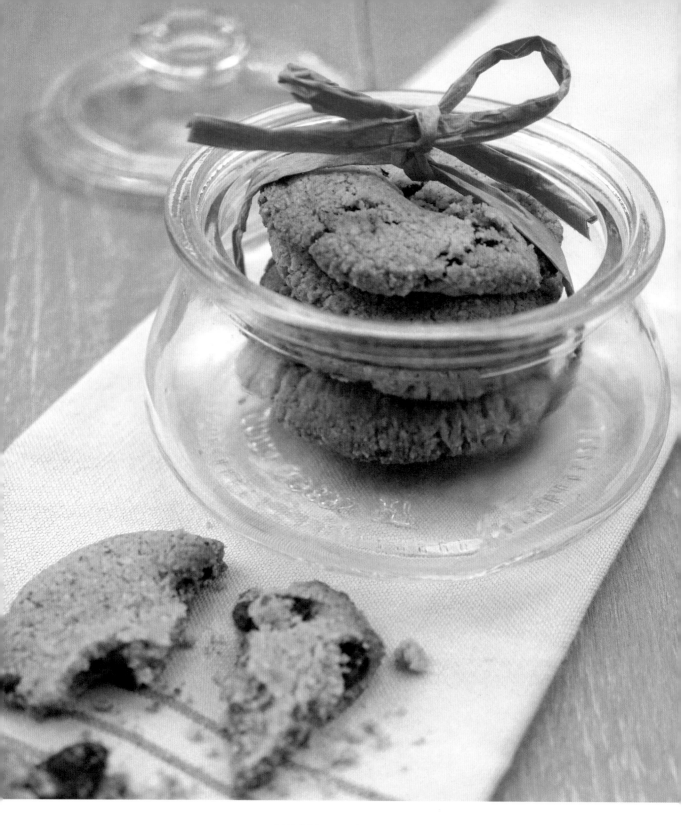

Cinnamon cookies

with raisins

125g (4½oz) ground almonds
½ tsp bicarbonate of soda
½ vanilla pod
1 tsp ground cinnamon
1–2 tsp low-calorie sweetener
  such as Stevia
60g (2oz) soft butter
1 tbsp raisins

Preheat the oven to 190°C (375°F/Gas 5). Line a baking tray with baking parchment.

Combine the almonds and bicarbonate of soda in a bowl. Cut open the vanilla pod lengthways and scrape out the seeds with a small knife.

Add the vanilla seeds, cinnamon, sweetener, and butter to the almond mixture and mix together well. Finally work in the raisins.

Create 12 balls from the mixture, place these on the baking parchment, and press flat. Bake the cookies in the centre of the oven for 10–15 minutes, until golden. Remove from the tray and leave to cool on a wire rack. The cinnamon cookies will keep for several days stored in an airtight container.

At home	At work	Serves	Kcal	Protein	Carbs	Fat
10 + 15 mins	0 min	12	110	3g	2g	10g

Index

About the authors

We love healthy eating and for several years we have run a large food website discussing low-carb nutrition. At our website lowcarbrezepte.org you will find lots of delicious recipes, interesting contributions, and tips about the low-carb diet. We are passionate about creating new and delicious low-carb recipe ideas. When it comes to photographing the food, we believe in taking pictures that reflect how the food will actually be eaten.

Our recipes contain plenty of healthy ingredients to introduce variety to the snacks and meals you eat when you are on the go. We love real food and work mainly with ingredients that are unprocessed and good for our bodies. Our low-carb dishes are easy for the body to digest, which means that after lunch you can continue working at your very best, without any dips in concentration — the great thing about these low-carb recipes is that they don't make you sluggish and weary after eating and you won't get that craving to have a catnap under your desk.

The *Low Carb on the Go* cook book is designed for anyone wanting to follow a low-carb diet. The consumption of healthy, complex carbohydrates is crucial for well-functioning organs and vital for our health and wellbeing. We also want to encourage you to incorporate your own ideas. There's more than one way to approach things. Each of us has our own ideas and preferences — and quite right, too. That is why a recipe should never be regarded as set in stone, and there is no need to follow everything to the letter. You can and should adapt and improve the recipes according to your own preferences.

Ideally the low-carb approach will shape your nutritional intake in the long term and become a natural choice, rather than being a short-term diet in which you consciously avoid bad carbohydrates such as sugar, white flour, fast food, ready-made products, too many pastries, baked goods, and other unhealthy foods. Look after yourself by providing your body with healthy foods.

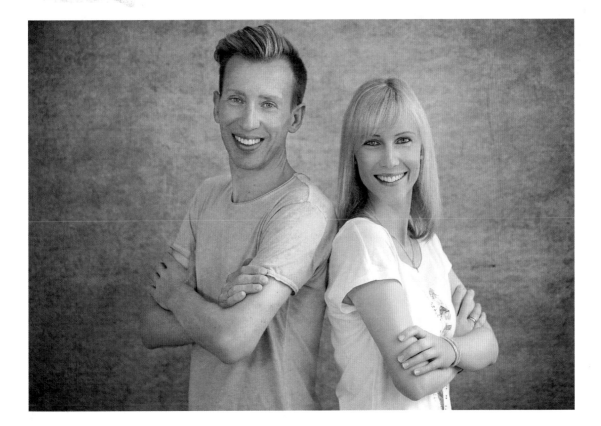

One final useful tip: treat yourself now and again to a "break" from the low-carb approach. Completely avoiding all wicked ingredients rarely achieves the desired effect. Every so often you should be able to choose a dish that doesn't entirely meet the low-carb rules. Choose your treat thoughtfully and enjoy every mouthful, then you can continue with your low-carb diet.

This way, you won't end up feeling like you have to completely miss out, or that certain foods are banned.

We hope you really enjoy our recipes.

Thank you

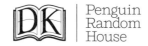

Text and photography Sandra and Mirco Stupning
Editor Karin Kerber
Designer Studio Rio, München

For DK Germany
Publisher Monika Schlitzer
Managing Editor Caren Hummel
Project Manager Melanie Haizmann
Production Manager Dorothee Whittaker
Production Coordinator Arnika Marx
Production Sabine Hüttenkofer, Verena Marquart
Author photo page 191 Julia Reinke

For DK UK
Translator Alison Tunley
Editor Claire Cross
Senior Editor Kathryn Meeker
Senior Art Editor Glenda Fisher
Producer, Pre-production Robert Dunn
Producer Igrain Roberts
Creative Technical Support Sonia Charbonnier
Managing Editor Stephanie Farrow
Managing Art Editor Christine Keilty

First British Edition, 2018
Dorling Kindersley Limited
80 Strand, London, WC2R 0RL
A Penguin Random House company

A CIP catalogue record for this book
is available from the British Library.
ISBN: 978-0-2413-4018-9

Printed and bound in China

A WORLD OF IDEAS:
SEE ALL THERE IS TO KNOW

www.dk.com